SZYCHER'S DICTIONARY
of
MEDICAL DEVICES

Michael Szycher, Ph.D.

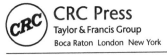

CRC Press
Taylor & Francis Group
Boca Raton London New York

CRC Press is an imprint of the
Taylor & Francis Group, an **informa** business

Szycher's Dictionary of Medical Devices
a TECHNOMIC publication

CRC Press
Taylor & Francis Group
6000 Broken Sound Parkway NW, Suite 300
Boca Raton, FL 33487-2742

First issued in paperback 2019

© 1995 by Taylor & Francis Group, LLC
CRC Press is an imprint of Taylor & Francis Group, an Informa business

No claim to original U.S. Government works

ISBN-13: 978-1-56676-275-5 (hbk)
ISBN-13: 978-0-367-40177-1 (pbk)

Library of Congress Catalog Card No. 95-60052

Visit the Taylor & Francis Web site at
http://www.taylorandfrancis.com

and the CRC Press Web site at
http://www.crcpress.com

To my wonderful wife, Laurie, whose unwavering support allows me the time to pursue all my professional activities, which included researching and writing this book. I am also privileged to share the joy of this new publication with my sons, Mark and Scott.

PREFACE

The field of medical devices represents one of the most advanced technological areas in the United States. In 1991, over 12 million Americans had at least one medical device; fixation devices had the highest incidence, followed by contact lens use and lens implants and, lastly, artificial joints. The public has come to expect that medical devices will alleviate maladies and/or conditions that were not treatable fifty years ago.

It is hard to believe that the first pacemaker was invented in the 1950s, the first artificial heart valve in 1952, and the first artificial hip replacement was performed in 1954. In 1992, the medical device industry exported a total of $6.9 billion, while the country imported a total of $3.9 billion, representing a $3.0 billion trade surplus.

Medical devices are among the most regulated products in the world. The FDA maintains a constant vigil over medical device manufacturers and importers; even medical device definitions are subject to official scrutiny. Title 21 of the Code of Federal Regulations publishes these definitions, but the definitions are spread over several medical specialty areas and are, thus, difficult to find. This book attempts to bring a measure of order by providing an alphabetical listing of officially defined devices.

The reader will find this dictionary a perfect companion to *Szycher's Dictionary of Biomaterials and Medical Devices*, which is also published by Technomic Publishing Co., Inc.

Abdominal Decompression Chamber A hoodlike Class III device used to reduce pressure on the pregnant patient's abdomen for the relief of abdominal pain during pregnancy or labor.

Abnormal Hemoglobin Assay A Class II device consisting of the reagents, apparatus, instrumentation, and controls necessary to isolate and identify abnormal genetically determined hemoglobin types.

Abrasive Disk A Class I device constructed of various abrasives, such as diamond chips, that are glued to shellac-based paper. The device is used to remove excessive restorative material, such as gold, and to smooth rough surfaces from oral restoration, such as crowns. The device is attached to a shank that is held by a handpiece.

Abrasive Point A Class I device used to remove excessive restorative material, such as gold, and to remove rough surfaces on oral restorations, such as amalgam fillings. The device may be constructed of diamond or silica particles molded into different shapes and fused to a shank that is held by a handpiece.

Abrasive Polishing Agent A Class I device in paste or powder form that contains an abrasive material, such as silica pumice, and is used to remove debris from the teeth. The abrasive polish is applied by a handpiece attachment (prophylaxis cup).

Absorbable Implant (Scleral buckling method) A Class II device intended to be implanted on the sclera to aid retinal reattachment.

Absorbable Poly(glycolide/L-lactide) Surgical Suture A Class II device composed of an absorbable sterile, flexible strand as prepared and synthesized from homopolymers of glycolide and co-polymers made from 90 percent glycolide and 10 percent lactide, and is indicated for use in soft tissue approximation. A PGL suture meets *United States Pharmacopeia* (U.S.P.) requirements as described in the U.S.P. "Monograph for Absorbable Surgical Sutures." It may be monofilament or multifilament (braided) in form, uncoated or coated, undyed or dyed with an FDA-approved color additive. Also, the suture may be provided with or without a standard needle attached.

Absorbable Powder for Lubricating a Surgeon's Glove A Class III device composed of powder made from cornstarch that meets the specifications for absorbable powder in the *United States Pharmacopeia* (U.S.P.) and that is intended to be used to lubricate the surgeon's hand before putting on a surgeon's glove. The device is absorbable through biological degradation.

Absorbable Surgical Gut Suture A Class II device, both plain and chromic, that is composed of an absorbable, sterile, flexible thread prepared from either the serosal connective tissue layer of beef (bovine) or the submucosal fibrous tissue of sheep (ovine) intestine, and is intended for use in soft-tissue approximation.

AC-Powered Adjustable Hospital Bed A Class II device consisting of a bed with a built-in electric motor and remote controls that can be operated by the patient to adjust the height and surface contour of the bed. The device includes movable and latchable side rails.

AC-Powered Bone Saw A Class II device with a serrated edge that is used during oral surgery for cutting and contouring bone.

AC-Powered Dental Amalgamator A Class II electrically powered device used to mix, by shaking, amalgam capsules containing mercury and dental alloy particles such as silver, tin, zinc, and copper. The resulting amalgam material is used for filling dental caries.

AC-Powered Dynamometer A Class II device intended for medical purposes to assess neuromuscular function, or degree of neuromuscular blockage, by measuring, with a force transducer (a device that translates force into electrical impulses), the grip-strength of a patient's hand.

AC-Powered Magnet A Class II device that generates a magnetic field intended to find and remove metallic foreign bodies from eye tissue.

AC-Powered Photostimulator A Class II device intended to provide light stimulus that allows measurement of retinal or visual function by perceptual or electrical methods (e.g., stroboscope).

AC-Powered Slitlamp Biomicroscope A Class II device that is a microscope intended for use in eye examination that projects into a patient's eye through a control diaphragm a thin, intense beam of light.

Acacia, Karaya Gum and Sodium Borate Denture Adhesive A Class III device that is applied to the base of a denture before the denture is inserted into the patient's mouth. The device is used to improve denture retention and comfort. There is a lack of information concerning the safety of adhesives containing sodium borate. Sodium borate concentration of 12–20 percent of the adhesive's total weight is equivalent to 2.6–5.3 percent boron. Because a portion of a dental adhesive is ingested, this amount of boron could cause chronic toxicity in denture wearers.

Acetaminophen Test System A Class II device intended to measure acetaminophen, an analgesic and fever reducing drug, in serum. Measurements obtained by this device are used in the diagnosis and treatment of acetaminophen overdose.

Acid Phosphatase (Total or prostatic) Test System A Class II device intended to measure the activity of the acid phosphatase enzyme in plasma and serum.

Acinetobacter calcoaceticus **Serological Reagents** Class I devices that consist of *Acinetobacter calcoaceticus* antigens and antisera used to identify this bacterium from cultured isolates derived from clinical specimens. The identification aids in the diagnosis of disease caused by the bacterium *Acinetobacter calcoaceticus* and provides epidemiological information on disease caused by this microorganism. This organism becomes pathogenic in patients with burns or with immunologic deficiency, and infection can result in sepsis (blood poisoning).

Acoustic Chamber for Audiometric Testing A Class I device, a room, that is intended for use in conducting diagnostic hearing evaluations and that eliminates sound reflections and provides isolation from outside sounds.

Act The Federal Food, Drug, and Cosmetic Act, as amended [secs. 201–902, 52 Stat. 1040 et seq., as amended (21 U.S.C. 321–392)].

Activated Whole Blood Clotting Time Test A Class II device used to monitor heparin therapy for the treatment of venous thrombosis or pulmonary embolism, and therapy for deficiencies of coagulation factors VIII (antihemophilic factor), IX (plasma thromboplastin component), and XI (plasma thromboplastin antecedent), by measuring the coagulation time of whole blood.

Adapter [Short Increment Sensitivity Index (SISI) adapter] A Class I device used with an audiometer in diagnostic hearing evaluations. A SISI adapter provides short periodic sound pulses in specific small decibel increments that are intended to be superimposed on the audiometer's output tone frequency.

Adaptometer (Biophotometer) An AC-powered Class I device that provides a stimulating light source that has various controlled intensities intended to measure the time required for retinal adaptation (regeneration of the visual purple) and the minimum light threshold.

Adenine Nucleotide Assay A Class I device that measures the levels in the body tissues and fluids of adenine nucleotide (a compound consisting of the base adenine, a sugar, and a phosphate group). This measurement is often made with a photometer (a device that measures light intensity) Adenosine diphosphate (ADP) is the nucleotide responsible for platelet aggregation in the arrest of bleeding.

Adenovirus Serological Reagents Class I devices that consist of antigens and antisera that are used in serological tests to identify adenovirus antibodies in a patient's serum. Additionally, some of these reagents consist of adenovirus antisera conjugated with a fluorescent dye and are used to identify adenoviruses directly from clinical specimens. The identification aids in the diagnosis of diseases caused by adenovirus infections and provides epidemiological information on these diseases. Adenovirus infections may cause pharyngitis (inflammation of the throat), acute respiratory diseases, and certain external diseases of the eye (e.g., conjunctivitis).

Adhesive (Drape adhesive)   A Class I device intended to be placed on the skin to attach a surgical drape.

Adhesive (External prosthesis adhesive)   A Class I device composed of a silicone-type adhesive intended to be used to fasten to the body an external aesthetic restoration prosthesis, such as an artificial nose.

Adhesive Tape and Bandage   A Class I device that consists of a strip of material or plastic, coated on one side with an adhesive, and may include a pad of surgical dressing without a disinfectant. The device is used to cover and protect wounds, to hold together the skin edges of a wound, to support an injured part of the body, and to secure objects to the skin.

Adrenocorticotropic Hormone (ACTH) Test System   A Class II device intended to measure adrenocorticotropic hormone in plasma and serum. ACTH measurements are used in the differential diagnosis and treatment of certain disorders of the adrenal glands such as Cushing's syndrome, adrenocortical insufficiency, and the ectopic ACTH syndrome.

Aerator Cabinet   A Class II device consisting of a cabinet equipped with a ventilator system designed to circulate and exchange the air contained in the cabinet to remove residual ethylene oxide gas following sterilization.

Afterimage Flasher   An AC-powered Class II device composed of a light that automatically switches on and off to allow performance of an afterimage test in which the patient indicates the positions of afterimages after the light is off. The device is intended to determine harmonious/anomalous retinal correspondence (the condition in which corresponding points on the retina have the same directional value).

Air Brush   A Class III AC-powered device used in conjunction with articulation paper. The device uses air-driven particles to roughen the surfaces of dental restorations; uneven areas of the restorations are then identified by use of articulation paper.

Air Fluidized Bed   A Class II device employing the circulation of filtered air through ceramic spherules (small round ceramic objects) to treat decubitus ulcers (bedsores), severe and extensive burns, and aid circulation.

Air or Water Caloric Stimulator A Class I device that delivers a stream of air or water to the ear canal at controlled rates of flow and temperature and that is intended for vestibular function testing of a patient's body balance system. The vestibular stimulation of the semicircular canals produces involuntary eye movements that are measured and recorded by a nystagmograph.

Air or Water Syringe Unit A Class I device that is used for the irrigation or drying of tooth or gum tissue. It consists of a tube to deliver air or water to the patient's mouth. The device may be attached to a dental operative unit.

Air-Handling Apparatus for a Surgical Operating Room A Class II device intended to produce a directed, nonturbulent flow of air that has been filtered to remove particulate matter and microorganisms to provide an area free of contaminants to reduce the possibility of infection in the patient.

Airway A Class II device inserted into the pharynx through the mouth to provide a patent airway.

Airway Connector A Class II device used to connect a breathing-gas source to a tracheal tube, tracheotomy tube or mask.

Airway, Nasopharyngeal A Class II device used to facilitate breathing by means of a tube inserted into the pharynx through the nose to provide a patient with an airway.

Alanine Amino Transferase (ALT/SGPT) Test System A Class I device intended to measure the activity of the enzyme alanine amino transferase (ALT) (also known as a serum glutamic pyruvic transaminase or SGPT) in serum and plasma. Alanine amino transferase measurements are used in the diagnosis and treatment of certain liver diseases (e.g., viral hepatitis and cirrhosis) and heart diseases.

Albumin Immunological Test System A Class II device that consists of the reagents used to measure, by immunochemical techniques, the albumin (a plasma protein) in serum and other body fluids. Measurement of albumin aids in the diagnosis of kidney and intestinal diseases.

Albumin Test System A Class II device intended to measure the albumin concentration in serum and plasma. Albumin measurements are used in the diagnosis and treatment of numerous diseases involving primarily the liver or kidneys.

Alcohol Test System A device intended to measure alcohol (e.g., ethanol, methanol, isopropanol, etc.) in human body fluids (e.g., serum, whole blood, and urine). Measurements obtained by this device are used in the diagnosis and treatment of alcohol intoxication and poisoning.

Aldose Test System A Class I device intended to measure the activity

5

of the enzyme aldolase in serum or plasma. Aldolase measurements are used in the diagnosis and treatment of the early stages of acute hepatitis and for certain muscle diseases such as progressive Duchenne-type muscular dystrophy.

Aldosterone Test System   A Class II device intended to measure the hormone aldosterone in serum and urine. Aldosterone measurements are used in the diagnosis and treatment of primary aldosteronism (a disorder caused by the excessive secretion of aldosterone by the adrenal gland), hypertension caused by primary aldosteronism, selective hypoaldosteronism, edematous states, and other conditions of electrolyte imbalance.

Algesimeter   see MANUAL ALGESIMETER; POWERED ALGESIMETER.

Alkaline Phosphatase or Isoenzymes Test System   A Class II device intended to measure alkaline phosphatase or its isoenzymes (a group of enzymes with similar biological activity) in serum or plasma. Measurements of alkaline phosphatase or its isoenzymes are used in the diagnosis and treatment of liver, bone, parathyroid, and intestinal diseases.

Amalgam Alloy   A Class II device that consists of a metallic substance that is mixed with mercury to form filling material for dental caries.

Amikacin Test System   A Class II device intended to measure amikacin, an aminoglycoside antibiotic drug, in serum and plasma. Measurements obtained by this device are used in the diagnosis and treatment of amikacin overdose and in monitoring levels of amikacin to ensure appropriate therapy.

δ-Aminolevulinic Acid Test System   A Class I device intended to measure the level of δ-aminolevulinic acid (a precursor of porphyrin) in urine. δ-aminolevulinic acid measurements are used in the diagnosis and treatment of lead poisoning and certain porphyrias (diseases affecting the liver, gastrointestinal, and nervous systems that are accompanied by increased urinary excretion of various heme compounds including δ-aminolevulinic acid).

Ammonia Test System   A device intended to measure ammonia levels in blood, serum, and plasma. Ammonia measurements are used in the diagnosis and treatment of severe liver disorders, such as cirrhosis, hepatitis, and Reye's syndrome.

Amniotic Fluid Sampler (Amniocentesis tray)   A Class II device used for amniocentesis (transabdominal aspiration of fluid from the amniotic sac). The sampler consists of disposable instruments, drapes, specimen container, and other accessories, on a tray.

Amphetamine Test System   A Class II device intended to measure amphetamine, a central nervous system stimulating drug, in plasma and urine. Measurements obtained by this device are used in the diagnosis and treatment of amphetamine use or overdose and in the monitoring levels of amphetamine to ensure appropriate therapy.

Amsler Grid A Class I device composed of a series of charts with grids of different sizes that are held at 30 centimeters distance from the patient and intended to rapidly detect central and paracentral irregularities in the visual field.

Amylase Test System A Class II device intended to measure the activity of the enzyme amylase in serum and urine. Amylase measurements are used primarily for the diagnosis and treatment of pancreatitis (inflammation of the pancreas).

Anaerobic Chamber A Class I device intended to maintain an anaerobic (oxygen free) environment for the isolation and cultivation of anaerobic microorganisms, and is used in the diagnosis of disease.

Analyzer *see* ARGON GAS ANALYZER; BLOOD CARBON MONOXIDE ANALYZER (NONINDWELLING); BLOOD OXYHEMOGLOBIN CONCENTRATION ANALYZER (NONINDWELLING); BLOOD CARBON DIOXIDE PARTIAL PRESSURE ANALYZER (NONINDWELLING); BLOOD HYDROGEN ION CONCENTRATION ANALYZER (NONINDWELLING); BLOOD NITROGEN PARTIAL PRESSURE ANALYZER (NONINDWELLING); BLOOD OXYGEN PARTIAL PRESSURE ANALYZER (NONINDWELLING).

Androstenedione Test System A Class I device intended to measure androstenedione (a substance secreted by the testes, ovary, and adrenal glands) in serum. Adrostenedione measurements are used in the diagnosis and treatment of females with excessive levels of androgen (male sex hormone) production.

Androsterone Test System A Class I device intended to measure the hormone androsterone in serum, plasma, and urine. Androsterone measurements are used in the diagnosis and treatment of gonadal and adrenal diseases.

Anesthesia Breathing Circuit A Class II device used to administer medical gases during anesthesia. It provides both an inhalation and exhalation route and may include a connector, adaptor, and Y-piece.

Anesthesia Conduction Catheter A Class II device used to inject local anesthetics to provide continuous regional anesthesia.

Anesthesia Conduction Filter A Class II device composed of a microporous filter used while administering injections of local anesthetics to minimize particulate contamination of the injected fluid.

Anesthesia Conduction Kit A Class II device used to administer conduction anesthesia. The kit may contain syringes, needles and drugs.

Anesthesia Conduction Needle A Class II device used to inject local anesthetics to provide regional anesthesia.

Anesthesia Gas Machine A Class II device used to administer, continuously or intermittently, a general inhalation agent to maintain ventilation. The device may include gas flowmeter, vaporizer, ventilator, breathing circuit with bag, and emergency gas supply.

Anesthesia Stool A Class II device used as a stool for the anesthesiologist in the operating room.

Anesthetic Cabinet, Table or Tray A Class II device used to store anesthetic equipment and drugs. The device is usually constructed to eliminate build-up of static electrical charges.

Anesthetic Gas Mask A Class II device, usually made of conductive rubber, that is positioned over a patient's nose or mouth to direct anesthetic gases to the upper airway.

Anesthetic Vaporizer A Class II device used to vaporize liquid anesthetic and deliver a controlled amount of the vapor to the patient.

Anesthetic Warmer A Class II AC-powered device into which tubes containing anesthetic solution are placed in order to warm them prior to the administration of the anesthetic.

Angiographic Injector and Syringe A Class II device that consists of a syringe and a high-pressure injector which are used to inject contrast material into the heart, great vessels, and coronary arteries to study the heart and vessels by X-ray photography.

Angiographic X-ray System A Class II device intended for radiologic visualization of the heart, blood vessels, or lymphatic system during or after injection of a contrast medium. This generic type of device may include signal analysis and display equipment, patient and equipment supports, component parts, and accessories.

Angiotensin Converting Enzyme (ACE) Test System A Class II device intended to measure the activity of angiotensin converting enzyme in serum and plasma. Measurements obtained by this device are used in the diagnosis and treatment of diseases such as sarcoidosis, a disease characterized by the formation of nodules in the lungs, bones and skin, and Gaucher's disease, a hereditary disorder affecting the spleen.

Angiotensin I and Renin Test System A Class II device intended to measure the level of angiotensin I generated by renin in plasma. Angiotensin I measurements are used in the diagnosis and treatment of certain types of hypertension.

Animal and Human Sera Class I biological products, obtained from the blood of humans or other animals, that provide the necessary growth promoting nutrients in a cell culture system.

Ankle Joint Metal/Composite Semiconstrained Cemented Prosthesis A Class II device intended to be implanted to replace an ankle joint. The device limits translation and rotation in one or more planes via the geometry of its articulating surfaces. It has no linkage across-the-joint. This generic type of device includes prostheses that consist of a talar resurfacing component made of alloys, such as cobalt-chromium-molybdenum, and a tibial resurfacing component fabricated from ultra-high molecular weight polyethylene with carbon fiber composite, and is limited to those prostheses intended for use with bone cement.

Ankle Joint Metal/Polymer Nonconstrained Cemented Prosthesis A Class III device intended to be implanted to replace an ankle joint. The device limits minimally (less than normal anatomic constraints) translation in one or more planes. It has no linkage across-the-joint. This generic type of device includes prostheses that have a tibial component made of alloys, such as cobalt-chromium-molybdenum, and a talar component made of ultra-high molecular weight polyethylene, and is limited to those prostheses intended for use with bone cement.

Ankle Joint Metal/Polymer Semiconstrained Cemented Prosthesis A Class II device intended to be implanted to replace an ankle joint. The device limits translation and rotation in one or more planes via the geometry of its articulating surfaces and has no linkage across-the-joint. This generic type of device includes prostheses that have a talar resurfacing component made of alloys, such as cobalt-chromium-molybdenum, and a tibial resurfacing component made of ultra-high molecular weight polyethylene and is limited to those prostheses intended for use with bone cement.

Annuloplasty Ring A Class III device that is a rigid or flexible ring implanted around the mitral or tricuspid heart valve for reconstructive treatment of valvular insufficiency.

Anomaloscope An AC-powered Class I device intended to test for anomalies of color vision by displaying mixed spectral lines to be matched by the patient.

Antimicrobial Susceptibility Test Disk A Class II device that consists of antimicrobial-impregnated paper disks used to measure, by a disk-agar diffusion technique or a disk-broth elution technique, the in vitro susceptibility of most clinically important bacterial pathogens to antimicrobial agents. In the disk-agar diffusion technique, bacterial susceptibility is ascertained by directly measuring the magnitude of a zone of bacterial inhibition around the disk on an agar surface. The disk-broth elution technique is associated with an automated rapid susceptibility test system and employs a fluid medium in which susceptibility is ascertained by photometrically measuring changes in bacterial growth resulting when antimicrobial material is eluted from the disk into the fluid medium. Test results are used in the treatment of bacterial diseases to determine the antimicrobial agent of choice.

Antimicrobial Susceptibility Test Powder   A Class II device that consists of an antimicrobial drug powder packaged in vials in specified amounts and intended for use in clinical laboratories for determining in vitro susceptibility of bacterial pathogens to these therapeutic agents. Test results are used in the treatment of bacterial diseases to determine the antimicrobial agent of choice.

Antimitochondrial Antibody Immunological Test System   A Class II device that consists of the reagents used to measure, by immunochemical techniques, antimitochondrial antibodies in human serum. The measurements aid in the diagnosis of diseases that produce a spectrum of autoantibodies (antibodies produced against the body's own tissue) such as primary biliary cirrhosis (degeneration of liver tissue) and chronic active hepatitis (inflammation of the liver).

Antimony Test System   A Class I device intended to measure antimony, a heavy metal, in urine, blood, vomitus, and stomach contents. Measurements obtained by this device are used in the diagnosis and treatment of antimony poisoning.

Antinuclear Antibody Immunological Test System   A Class II device that consists of the reagents used to measure, by immunochemical techniques, the autoimmune antibodies in serum and tissues that react with cellular nuclear constituents (molecules present in the nucleus of a cell, such as ribonucleic acid, deoxyribonucleic acid, or nuclear proteins) in serum or body fluids. The measurements aid in the diagnosis of systemic lupus erythematosus, a multisystem autoimmune disease (a disease in which antibodies attack the victim's own tissues), hepatitis (a liver disease), rheumatoid arthritis, Sjogren's syndrome (arthritis with inflammation of the eye, eyelid, and salivary glands) and systemic sclerosis (chronic hardening and shrinking of many body tissues).

Antiparietal Antibody Immunological Test System   A Class II device that consists of the reagents used to measure, by immunochemical techniques, the specific antibody for gastric parietal cells in human serum and body fluids. Gastric parietal cells are those cells located in the stomach that produce a protein that enables vitamin B_{12} to be absorbed by the body. The measurements aid in the diagnosis of vitamin B_{12} deficiency (or pernicious anemia) atrophic gastritis (inflammation of the stomach), and autoimmune connective tissue diseases (diseases resulting when the body produces antibodies against its own tissues).

Antismooth Muscle Antibody Immunological Test System   A Class II device that consists of the reagents used to measure, by immunochemical techniques, the antismooth muscle antibodies (antibodies to nonstriated, involuntary muscle) in serum. The measurements aid in the diagnosis of chronic hepatitis (inflammation of the liver) and autoimmune connective tissue diseases (diseases resulting from antibodies produced against the body's own tissues).

Antistammering Device   A Class I device that electronically generates a noise when activated or when it senses the user's speech. It is intended to prevent the user from hearing the sound of his or her own voice. The device is used to minimize a user's involuntary hesitative or repetitive speech.

Antithrombin III Assay   A Class II device that is used to determine the plasma level of antithrombin III (a substance that acts with the anticoagulant heparin to prevent coagulation). This determination is used to monitor the administration of heparin in the treatment of thrombosis. The determination may also be used in the diagnosis of thrombophilia (a congenital deficiency of antithrombin III).

Antitrypsin Immunological Test System   A device that consists of the reagents used to measure, by immunochemical techniques, the α-1-antitrypsin (a plasma protein) in serum, tissue, and other body fluids. The measurements aid in the diagnosis of several conditions including juvenile and adult cirrhosis of the liver. In addition, α-1-antitrypsin deficiency has been associated with pulmonary emphysema.

Apex Cardiograph (Vibrocardiograph)   A Class II device used to amplify or condition the signal from an apex cardiographic transducer and to produce a visual display of the motion of the heart. This device also provides any excitation energy required by the transducer.

Apex Cardiographic Transducer   A Class II device used to detect motion of the heart (acceleration, velocity or displacement) by changes in the mechanical or electrical properties of the device.

Argon Gas Analyzer   A Class II diagnostic anesthesiology device used to measure the connection of argon gas in a gas mixture used to determine the ventilatory status of a patient. The device may use techniques such as mass spectrometry or thermal conductivity for gas analysis.

***Arizona* spp. Serological Reagents**   Class I devices that consist of antisera and antigens used to identify *Arizona* spp. in cultured isolates derived from clinical specimens. The identification aids in the diagnosis of disease caused by bacteria belonging to the genus *Arizona* and provides epidemiological information on diseases caused by these microorganisms. *Arizona* spp. can cause gastroenteritis (food poisoning) and sepsis (blood poisoning).

Arm Sling   A Class I device used to immobilize the arm by means of a fabric band suspended from around the neck.

Arrhythmia Detector and Alarm A Class III device that monitors the electrocardiogram (ECG) and is designed to produce a visible or audible signal or alarm when an atrial or ventricular arrhythmia exists, such as premature contraction or ventricular fibrillation.

Arsenic Test System A Class I device intended to measure arsenic, a poisonous heavy metal, in urine, vomitus, stomach contents, nails, hair, and blood. Measurements obtained by this device are used in the diagnosis and treatment of arsenic poisoning.

Arterial Blood Sampling Kit A Class II diagnostic anesthesiology device, in kit form, used to acquire arterial blood samples for blood gas determinations, such as arterial oxygen tension. The kit usually contains a syringe, needle, cork and heparin anticoagulant.

Arthroscope An electrically powered Class II device composed of an endoscope intended to make visible the interior of a joint. The arthroscope and accessories are also intended to perform surgery within a joint.

Articulation Paper A Class I device composed of paper coated with an ink dye that is placed between the upper and lower teeth when the teeth are in the bite position. The articulation paper is used to locate uneven or high areas.

Articulator A Class I mechanical device used to simulate movements of a patient's upper and lower jaw. Plaster casts of the patient's teeth and gums are placed in the device to reproduce the occlusion (bite) and articulation of the patient's jaws. An articulator is used to fit dentures or provide orthodontic treatment.

Artificial Eye A Class II device resembling an eyeball, usually made of glass or plastic, intended to be inserted in a patient's eye socket for cosmetic purposes to replace an eye. The device is not intended to be implanted.

Ascorbic Acid Test System A Class II device intended to measure the level of ascorbic acid (vitamin C) in plasma, serum, and urine. Ascorbic acid measurements are used in the diagnosis and treatment of ascorbic acid dietary deficiencies.

Aspartate Amino Transferase (AST/SGOT) Test System A Class II device intended to measure the activity of the enzyme aspartate amino transferase (AST) (also known as a serum glutamic oxaloacetic transferase or SGOT) in serum and plasma. Aspartate amino transferase measurements are used in the diagnosis and treatment of certain types of liver and heart disease.

***Aspergillus* spp. Serological Reagents** Class I devices that consist of antigens and antisera used in various serological tests to identify *Aspergillus* spp. antibodies in a patient's serum. The identification aids in the diagnosis of aspergillosis caused by fungi belonging to the genus *Aspergillus*. Aspergillosis is a disease marked by inflammatory granulomatous (tumor-like) lesions in the skin, ear, eyeball cavity, nasal sinuses, lungs, and occasionally, the bones.

Atomic Absorption Spectrophotometer for Clinical Use   A Class I device intended to identify and measure elements and metals (e.g., lead and mercury) in human specimens. The metal elements are identified according to the wavelength and intensity of the light that is absorbed when the specimen is converted to the atomic vapor phase. Measurements obtained by this device are used in the diagnosis and treatment of certain conditions.

Audiometer (or Automated audiometer)   An electroacoustic Class II device that produces controlled levels of test tones and signals intended for use in conducting diagnostic hearing evaluations and assisting in the diagnosis of possible otologic disorders.

Audiometer Calibration Set   An electronic reference Class II device that is intended to calibrate an audiometer. It measures the sound frequency and intensity characteristics that emanate from an audiometer earphone. The device consists of an acoustic cavity of known volume, a sound level meter, a microphone with calibration traceable to the National Bureau of Standards, oscillators, frequency counters, microphone amplifiers, and a recorder. The device can measure selected audiometer test frequencies at a given intensity level, and selectable audiometer attenuation settings at a given test frequency.

Audit   A documented activity performed in accordance with written procedures on a periodic basis to verify, by examination and evaluation of objective evidence, compliance with those elements of the quality assurance program under review. "Audit" does not include surveillance or inspection activities performed for the purpose of conducting a quality assurance program or undertaking complaint investigations or failure analyses of a device.

Auditory Impedance Tester   A Class II device that is intended to change the air pressure in the external auditory canal and measure and graph the mobility characteristics of the tympanic membrane to evaluate the functional condition of the middle ear. The device is used to determine abnormalities in the mobility of the tympanic membrane due to stiffness, flaccidity, or the presence of fluid in the middle ear cavity. The device is also used to measure the acoustic reflex threshold from contractions of the stapedial muscle, to monitor healing of tympanic membrane grafts or stapedectomies, or to monitor follow-up treatment for inflammation of the middle ear.

Automated Blood Cell Diluting Apparatus   A Class I device used to make, automatically, appropriate dilutions of a blood sample for further quantitative testing.

Automated Blood Cell Separator   A Class III device that automatically removes whole blood from a donor, separates the blood into components (red blood cells, white blood cells, plasma, and platelets), retains one or more of the components, and returns the remainder of the blood to the donor. The components obtained are transfused or used to prepare blood products for administration.

Automated Blood Grouping and Antibody Test System   A Class II device used to group erythrocytes (red blood cells) and to detect antibodies to blood group antigens.

Automated Cell Counter   A Class II device used to count red blood cells, white blood cells, or blood platelets, to measure hemoglobin and hematocrit, and to measure or calculate the red cell indices (the erythrocyte mean corpuscular volume, the mean corpuscular hemoglobin, and the mean corpuscular hemoglobin concentration) using a sample of the patient's peripheral blood (blood circulating in one of the body's extremities, such as the arm.

Automated Cell Locating Device   A Class II device used to locate blood cells on a peripheral blood smear, allowing the operator to identify and classify each cell according to type. (Peripheral blood is blood circulating in one of the body's extremities, such as the arm.)

Automated Cell-Washing Centrifuge for Immuno-Hematology   A Class II device used to separate and prepare cells and sera for further in vitro diagnostic testing.

Automated Colony Counter   A mechanical Class I device used to determine the number of bacterial colonies present on a bacteriological culture medium contained in a petri plate. The number of colonies counted is used in the diagnosis of disease as a measure of the degree of bacterial infection.

Automated Coombs Test System   A Class II device used to detect and identify antibodies in patient sera or antibodies bound to red cells. The Coombs test is used for the diagnosis of hemolytic disease of the newborn and autoimmune hemolytic anemia. The test is also used in crossmatching and investigating transfusion reactions and drug-induced red cell sensitization.

Automated Differential Cell Counter   A Class III device used to identify and classify one or more of the formed elements of the blood.

Automated Hematocrit Instrument   A Class II device that measures automatically the packed red cell volume of a blood sample to distinguish normal from abnormal states, such as anemia and erythrocytosis (an increase in the number of red cells).

Automated Hemoglobin System   A Class II device consisting of the reagents, calibrators, controls, and instrumentation used to determine the hemoglobin content of human blood.

Automated Heparin Analyzer   A Class III device used to determine the heparin level in a blood sample by mixing the sample with prot-amine (a heparin neutralizing substance) and determining pho-tometrically the onset of air activated clotting. The analyzer also determines the amount of protamine necessary to neutralize the heparin in the patient's circulation.

Automated Medium Dispensing and Stacking Device A Class I mechanical device used to dispense a microbiological culture medium into petri dishes followed by the mechanical stacking of the petri dishes. This device aids in the diagnosis of disease.

Automated Platelet Aggregation System A Class II device used to determine changes in platelet shape and platelet aggregation follow-ing the addition of an aggregating reagent to a platelet-rich plasma.

Automated Sedimentation Rate Device A Class I device that measures automatically the erythrocyte sedimentation rate in whole blood. Because an increased sedimentation rate indicates tissue damage or inflammation, the erythrocyte sedimentation rate device is useful in monitoring treatment of a disease.

Automated Slide Spinner A Class II device that prepares automati-cally a blood film on a microscope slide using a small amount of peripheral blood (blood circulating in one of the body's extremities, such as the arm).

Automated Slide Strainer A Class I device used to stain histology, cytology, and hematology slides for diagnosis.

Automated Tissue Processor A Class I automated system used to process tissue specimens for examination through fixation, dehydration, and infiltration.

Automated Urinalysis System A device intended to measure certain of the physical properties and chemical constituents of urine by procedures that duplicate manual urinalysis systems. This device is used in conjunction with certain materials to measure a variety of urinary analytes.

Automated Zone Reader A mechanical Class I device used to measure zone diameters of microbial growth inhibition (or exhibi-tion), such as those observed on the surface of certain culture media used in disk-agar diffusion antimicrobial susceptibility tests. The device aids in the diagnosis of disease.

Automatic Catheter Flushing Device A Class II device used to pump fluid into an intravascular catheter to prevent clot formation.

Automatic Radiographic Film Processor A Class II device intended to be used to develop, fix, wash, and dry automatically and continu-ously film exposed for medical purposes.

Automatic Rotating Tourniquet A Class II device that prevents blood flow in one limb at a time, which temporarily reduces the total blood flow volume, thereby reducing the normal workload of the heart.

Autotransfusion Apparatus   A Class III device that consists of a roller pump, nylon mesh filter, reservoir, and auxiliary filter used to collect and reinfuse a patient's blood during surgery.

B

Bagolini Lens   A Class I device that consists of a plane lens containing almost imperceptible striations that do not obscure visualization of objects. The device is placed in a trial frame and is intended to determine harmonious/anomalous retinal correspondence (a condition in which corresponding points on the retina have the same directional values).

Balanced Salt Solutions or Formulations   A defined mixture of salts and glucose in a simple medium. This Class I device is included as a necessary component of most cell culture systems. This media component controls for pH, osmotic pressure, energy source, and inorganic ions.

Ballistocardiograph   A Class II device, including a supporting structure on which a patient is placed, that moves in response to blood ejected from the heart. The device usually includes a visual display.

Bandage (Adhesive tape and bandage)   A Class I device which consists of a strip of material or plastic, coated on one side with an adhesive, and may include a pad of surgical dressing without a disinfectant. The device is used to cover and protect wounds, to hold together the skin edges of a wound, to support an injured part of the body, and to secure objects to the skin.

Bandage, Elastic   A Class I device consisting of either a long, flat strip or a tube of elasticized material used to support or compress a part of the body.

Bandage, Liquid   A Class I device composed of a sterile liquid used to cover an opening in the skin or as a dressing for burns.

Barbiturate Test System   A Class II device intended to measure barbiturates, a class of hypnotic and sedative drugs, in serum, urine, and gastric contents. Measurements obtained by this device are used in the diagnosis and treatment of barbiturate use or overdose and in monitoring levels of barbiturate to ensure appropriate therapy.

Base Metal Alloy   A Class II device composed of a material, such as a mixture of nickel and chromium, that is used in the fabrication of a custom-made dental device, such as porcelain veneer for a tooth.

Battery-Powered Artificial Larynx An externally applied Class I device intended for use in the absence of the larynx to produce sound. When held against the skin in the area of the voicebox, the device generates mechanical vibrations which resonate in the oral and nasal cavities and can be modulated by the tongue and lips in a normal manner, thereby allowing this production of speech.

Bed (AC-powered adjustable hospital) A Class II device consisting of a bed with a built-in electric motor and remote controls that can be operated by the patient to adjust the height and surface contour of the bed. The device includes movable and latchable side rails.

Bed (Hydraulic adjustable hospital) A Class I device consisting of a bed with a hydraulic mechanism operated by an attendant to adjust the height and surface contour of the bed. The device includes movable and latchable side rails.

Bed (Manual adjustable hospital) A Class I device consisting of a bed with a manual mechanism operated by an attendant to adjust the height and surface contour of the bed. The device includes movable and latchable side rails.

Bence-Jones Proteins Immunological Test System A Class II device that consists of the reagents used to measure, by immunochemical techniques, the Bence-Jones proteins in urine and serum. Immunoglobulin molecules normally consist of pairs of polypeptide chains (subunits) of unequal size (light chains and heavy chains) bound together by several disulfide bridges. In some cancerous conditions there is a proliferation of one plasma cell (antibody-producing cell) with excess production of light chains of one specific kind (monoclonal light chains). These free homogeneous light chains not associated with an immunoglobulin molecule can be found in patient's plasma and urine, and have been called Bence-Jones proteins. Measurement of Bence-Jones proteins and determination that they are monoclonal aid in the diagnosis of multiple myeloma (malignant proliferation of plasma cells), Waldenstrom's macroglobulinemia (increased production of large immunoglobulins by spleen and bone marrow cells), leukemia (cancer of the blood forming organs), and lymphoma (cancer of the lymphoid tissue).

Benzodiazepine Test System A Class II device intended to measure any of the benzodiazepine compounds, sedative and hypnotic drugs, in blood, plasma, and urine. The benzodiazepine compounds include chlordiazepoxide, diazepam, oxazepam, chlorzepate, flurazepam, and nitrazepam. Measurements obtained by this device are used in the diagnosis and treatment of benzodiazepine use or overdose and in monitoring levels of benzodiazepines to ensure appropriate therapy.

Beta or Gamma Counter for Clinical Use A Class I device intended

17

to detect and count beta or gamma radiation emitted by clinical samples. Clinical samples are prepared by addition of a radioactive reagent to the sample. These measurements are useful in the diagnosis and treatment of various disorders.

Beta Globulin Immunological Test System   A Class I device that consists of the reagents used to measure, by immunochemical techniques, beta globulins (serum protein) in serum and other body fluids. Beta globulin proteins include beta lipoprotein, transferrin, glycoproteins, and complement and are rarely associated with specific pathological disorders.

Bicarbonate/Carbon Dioxide Test System   A Class II device intended to measure bicarbonate/carbon dioxide in plasma serum, and whole blood. Bicarbonate/carbon dioxide measurements are used in the diagnosis and treatment of numerous potentially serious disorders associated with changes in body acid-base balance.

Biliary Catheter and Accessories   A Class II tubular, flexible device used for temporary or prolonged drainage of the biliary tract, for splinting of the bile duct during healing, or for preventing stricture of the bile duct. This generic type of device may include a bile collecting bag that is attached to the biliary catheter by a connector and fastened to the patient with a strap.

Bilirubin (Total and unbound) in the Neonate Test System   A Class I device intended to measure the levels of bilirubin (total and unbound) in the blood (serum) of newborn infants to aid in indicating the risk of bilirubin encephalopathy (kernicterus).

Bilirubin (Total or direct) Test System   A Class II device intended to measure the levels of bilirubin (total or direct) in plasma or serum. Measurements of the levels of bilirubin (an organic compound formed during the normal and abnormal destruction of red blood cells), are used in the diagnosis and treatment of liver, hemolytic, hematological, and metabolic disorders, including hepatitis and gall bladder block.

Biofeedback Device   A Class II device that provides a signal corresponding to the status of the patient's physiological parameters (brain alpha waves, muscle activity, skin temperatue, etc.) so that the patient can voluntarily control these parameters.

Biopotential Amplifier and Signal Conditioner   A Class II device used to amplify or condition an electrical signal of biologic origin.

Biopsy Device   A Class II device used to remove samples of tissue for diagnostic purposes.

Biopsy Device, Endomyocardial   A Class II device used to remove samples of tissue from the inner wall of the heart.

Bipolar Endoscopic Coagulator-Cutter and Accessories A Class III device used to perform female sterilization and other operative procedures under endoscopic observation. It destroys tissue with high temperatures by directing a high frequency electrical current through tissue between two electrical contacts of a probe. This generic type of device includes the following accessories: an electrical generator, probes, and electrical cables.

***Blastomyces dermatitides* Serological Reagents** Class II devices that consist of antigens and antisera used in serological tests to identify the antibodies to *Blastomyces dermatitides* in a patient's serum. The identification aids in the diagnosis of blastomycosis caused by the fungus *Blastomyces dermatitides*. Blastomycosis is a chronic granulomatous (tumor-like) disease, which may be limited to the skin or lung or may be widely disseminated in the body resulting in lesions of the bones, liver, spleen, and kidneys.

Bleeding Time Device A Class II device, usually employing two spring-loaded blades that produce two small incisions in the skin. The length of time required for the bleeding to stop is a measure of the effectiveness of the coagulation system, particularly the platelets.

Blood Access Device A Class II device intended to provide access to the blood for hemodialysis or equivalent uses.

Blood Access Device and Accessories A Class II device intended to provide acess to a patient's blood for hemodialysis or substantially equivalent uses. When used for hemodialysis, it is part of an artificial kidney system for the treatment of patients with renal failure or toxemic conditions and provides access to a patient's blood for hemodialysis. The device includes implanted blood access devices and nonimplanted blood access devices and accessories. Accessories common to either type include the shunt adaptor, cannula clamp, shunt stabilizer, vessel dilator, disconnect forceps, shunt guard, crimp plier, tube plier, crimp ring, joint ring, fistula adaptor, and declotting tray (including accessories are either connected to a system, such as the hemodialysis system and during dialysis, or are plugged or connected together. This generic type of device includes various shunts and connectors specifically designed to provide access to blood, such as the arteriovenous shunt cannula and vessel tip. (1) The implanted blood access device consists of various flexible or rigid tubes, which are surgically implanted in appropriate blood vessels, and come through the skin, and are intended to remain in the body for thirty days or more. (2) The nonimplanted blood access device consists of various flexible or rigid tubes, such as catheters, cannulae or hollow needles, which are inserted into appropriate blood vessels or a vascular graft prosthesis and are intended to remain in the body for fewer than thirty days. This generic type of device includes fistula needles, the single needle dialysis set (coaxial flow needle), and the single needle dialysis set (alternating flow, needle only).

Blood Bank Centrifuge for in vitro Diagnostic Use   A Class I device used only to separate blood cells for further diagnostic testing.

Blood Bank Supplies   General purpose, Class I devices for, in vitro, use in blood banking. This generic type of device includes products such as blood bank pipettes, blood grouping slides, blood typing tubes, blood typing racks, and cold packs for antisera reagents. The device does not include articles that are licensed by FDA's Bureau of Biologics.

Blood Carbon Dioxide Partial Pressure Analyzer (Nonindwelling)   A Class II diagnostic anesthesiology device which is used to measure, in vitro, the partial pressure of carbon dioxide in blood, and is an aid in determining a patient's circulatory, ventilatory, and metabolic status. The device may use analytical techniques such as chemical titration, electrochemistry, or mass spectrometry.

Blood Carbon Monoxide Analyzer (Nonindwelling)   A Class II diagnostic anesthesiology device used to measure, in vitro, the concentration of carboxyhemoglobin (i.e., the decrease in oxygen-carrying capacity of hemoglobin) in blood, as an aid in determing a patient's physiological status.

Blood Cell Diluent   A Class I device used to dilute blood for further testing, such as blood cell counting.

Blood Gases (PCO$_2$, PO$_2$) and Blood pH Test System   A Class II device intended to measure certain gases in blood, serum, plasma or pH of blood, serum, and plasma. Measurements of blood gases (PCO$_2$, PO$_2$) and blood pH are used in the diagnosis and treatment of life-threatening acid-base disturbances.

Blood Group Substances of Nonhuman Origin for in vitro Diagnostic Use   Class I devices composed of materials, such as blood group specific substances prepared from nonhuman sources (e.g., pigs, cattle, and horses), used to detect, identify, or neutralize antibodies to various human blood group antigens. This generic type of device does not include materials that are licensed by FDA's Bureau of Biologics.

Blood Grouping View Box   A Class I device with a glass or plastic viewing surface, which may be illuminated and heated, that is used to view cell reactions in antigen-antibody testing.

Blood Hydrogen Ion Concentration Analyzer (Nonindwelling)   A Class II diagnostic anesthesiology device which is used to measure, in vitro, the hydrogen ion concentration (pH) of blood, and is an aid in determining the patient's acid-base balance.

Blood Mixing and Weighing Device   A Class I device used to mix blood or blood components by agitation or to weigh blood or blood components as they are collected.

Blood Nitrogen Partial Pressure Analyzer (Nonindwelling) A Class II diagnostic anesthesiology device which is used to measure, in vitro, the partial pressure of nitrogen (P_{N_2}), and is an aid in determining the patient's circulatory, ventilatory, and metabolic status.

Blood Oxygen Partial Pressure Analyzer (Nonindwelling) A Class II diagnostic anesthesiology device which is used to measure, in vitro, the partial pressure of oxygen (P_{O_2}), and is an aid in determining the patient's circulatory, ventilatory and metabolic status. The device may use analytical techniques such as electrochemical electrodes, gas chromatography, or mass spectrometry.

Blood Oxyhemoglobin Concentration Analyzer (Nonindwelling) A Class II diagnostic anesthesiology device which is used to measure, in vitro, the concentration of oxyhemoglobin (i.e., the oxygen-carrying capacity of hemoglobin) in blood, and is an aid in determining a patient's physiological status.

Blood and Plasma Warming Device A nonelectromagnetic Class III device that warms blood or plasma, by means other than electromagnetic radiation, prior to administration. An electromagnetic blood and plasma warming device is a device that employs electromagnetic radiation (radiowaves or microwaves) to warm a bag or bottle of blood or plasma prior to administration.

Blood Pressure Alarm A Class II device that accepts the signal from a blood pressure transducer amplifier, processes the signal, and emits an alarm when the blood pressure falls outside a preset upper or lower limit.

Blood Pressure Computer A Class II device that accepts the electrical signal from a blood pressure transducer amplifier and indicates the systolic, diastolic, or mean pressure based on the input signal.

Blood Pressure Cuff A Class II device that has an inflatable bladder in an inelastic sleeve (cuff) with a mechanism for inflating and deflating the bladder. The cuff is used in conjunction with another device to determine a subject's blood pressure.

Blood Pressure Management System A Class II device that provides a signal from which diastolic, systolic, mean, or any combination of the three can be derived through the use of transducers placed on the surface of the body.

Blood Specimen Collection Device A Class II device intended for medical purposes to collect and to handle blood specimens and to separate serum from nonserum (cellular) components prior to further testing. This generic type device may include blood collection tubes, vials, systems, serum separators, blood collection trays, or vacuum sample tubes.

Blood Storage Refrigerator and Blood Storage Freezer   Class II devices used to preserve blood and blood products by storing them at cold or freezing temperatures.

Blood Transfusion Microfilter   A Class II device used to remove microaggregates from blood or blood products during transfusion.

Blood Volume Measuring Device   A Class II device that is a manual, semiautomated, or automated system used to calculate the red cell mass, plasma volume, and total blood volume.

Blood Volume Test System   A Class I device intended to measure the circulating blood volume. Blood volume measurements are used in the diagnosis and treatment of stock, hemorrhage, and polycythemia vera (a disease characterized by an absolute increase in erythrocyte mass and total blood volume).

Blow Bottle   A Class I device used to induce a forced expiration from a patient. The patient blows into the device to move a column of water from one bottle to another.

Boiling Water Sterilizer   A Class I AC-powered device used to sterilize dental and surgical instruments by submersion of the instruments into boiling water.

Bone Cap   A mushroom-shaped Class II device intended to be implanted and made of either silicone elastomer or ultra-high molecular weight polyethylene. It is used to cover the severed end of a long bone such as the humerus or tibia, to control bone overgrowth in juvenile amputees.

Bone Densitometer   A Class II device intended for medical purposes to measure bone density and mineral content by X-ray or gamma ray transmission measurements through the bone and adjacent tissues. This generic type of device may include signal analysis and display equipment, patient and equipment supports, component parts, and accessories.

Bone Fixation Cerclage   A Class II device intended to be implanted that is made of alloys, such as cobalt-chromium-molybdenum, and that consists of a metallic ribbon or a flat sheet or a wire. The device is wrapped around the shaft of a long bone, anchored to the bone with wire or screws, and used in the fixation of fractures.

Bone Heterograft   A Class III device intended to be implanted that is made from mature (adult) bovine bones and used to replace human bone following surgery in the cervical region of the spinal column.

Bone Plate   A Class II metal device used to stabilize fractured bone structures in the oral cavity. The bone segments are attached to the plate with screws to prevent movement of the segments.

Bone Saw (AC-powered)   A Class II device with a serrated edge that is used during oral surgery for cutting and contouring bone. It is a device attached to a closed breathing circuit. The device is used to circulate anesthetic gases continuously by maintaining the unidirectional valves in an open position and reducing mechanical dead space and resistance in the breathing circuit.

Bordetella spp. Serological Reagents   Class I devices that consist of antigens and antisera, including antisera conjugated with a fluorescent dye, that are used in serological tests to identify *Bordetella* spp. from cultured isolates and/or directly from clinical specimens. The identification aids in the diagnosis of diseases caused by bacteria belonging to the genus *Bordetella* and provides epidemiological information on these diseases. *Bordetella* spp. cause whooping cough and other similarly contagious and acute respiratory infections characterized by pneumonitis (inflammation of the lungs).

Bothrop Atrox Reagent   A Class II device made from snake venom and used to determine blood fibrinogen levels to aid in the evaluation of disseminated intravascular coagulation (nonlocalized clotting in the blood vessels) in patients receiving heparin therapy (the administration of the anticoagulant heparin in the treatment of thrombosis) or as an aid in the classification of dysfibrinogenemia (presence in the plasma of functionally defective fibrinogen).

Bracket Adhesive Resin and Tooth Conditioner   A Class II device composed of an adhesive compound of polymethylmethacrylate that is used to cement an orthodontic bracket to a tooth surface.

Breast Milk Immunological Test System   A Class I device that consists of the reagents used to measure, by immunochemical techniques, the breast milk proteins.

Breath-Alcohol Test System   A Class I device intended to measure alcohol in the human breath. Measurements obtained by this device are used in the diagnosis of alcohol intoxication.

Breathing Circuit Bacterial Filter   A Class II device used to remove microbiological and particulate matter from the gases in the breathing circuit.

Breathing Circuit Circulator   A Class II device consisting of a turbine device attached to a closed breathing circuit. The device is used to circulate anesthetic gases continuously by maintaining the unidirectional valves in an open position and reducing mechanical dead space and resistance in the breathing circuit.

Breathing Gas Mixer   A Class II device used in conjunction with a respiratory support apparatus to facilitate and control the mixing of gases that are to be breathed by a patient.

Breathing Mouthpiece   A Class II device which is inserted into a patient's mouth that connects with diagnostic or therapeutic respiratory devices.

Breathing System Collection Bottle (Calibrated) A Class II calibrated breathing diagnostic anesthesiology device used to collect aspirated fluids from a patient, and capable of protecting the vacuum source by stopping the vacuum should the container overflow, thereby decreasing the risk of cross-patient infections.

Breathing System Collection Bottle (Uncalibrated) A Class I uncalibrated breathing diagnostic anesthesiology device used to collect aspirated fluids from a patient, and capable of protecting the vacuum source by stopping the vacuum should the container overflow, thereby decreasing the risk of cross-patient infections.

Breathing System Heater A Class II device used to warm respiratory gases before they enter the patient's airway. The device may include a temperature controller.

Breathing Tube Support A Class II device used to support and anchor a patient's breathing tube.

Bronchial Tube A Class II device used to differentially intubate a bronchus in order to isolate a portion of the lung distal to the tube.

Bronchoscope (Flexible or rigid) and Accessories A tubular endoscopic Class II device with any of a group of accessory devices which attach to the bronchoscope and is intended to examine or treat the larynx and tracheobronchial tree. It is typically used with a fiberoptic light source and carrier to provide illumination. The device is made of materials such as stainless steel or flexible plastic. This generic type of device includes the rigid ventilating bronchoscope, rigid nonventilating bronchoscope, nonrigid bronchoscope, laryngeal-bronchial telescope, flexible foreign body claw, bronchoscope tubing, flexible biopsy forceps, rigid biopsy curette, flexible biopsy brush, rigid biopsy forceps, flexible biopsy curette, and rigid bronchoscope aspirating tube, but excludes the fiberoptic light source and carrier.

***Brucella* spp. Serological Reagents** Class II devices that consist of antigens and antisera used for serological identification of *Brucella* spp. from cultured isolates derived from clinical specimens or to identify *Brucella* spp. antibodies in a patient's serum. Additionally, some of these reagents consist of antisera conjugated with a fluorescent dye (immunofluorescent reagents) used to identify *Brucella* spp. directly from clinical specimens and/or cultured isolates derived from clinical specimens. The identification aids in the diagnosis and treatment of brucellosis (e.g., undulant fever, Malta fever) caused by bacteria belonging to the genus *Brucella* and provides epidemiological information on disease caused by these microorganisms.

Burn Sheet A Class I device made of a porous material that is wrapped around a burn victim to provide warmth or barrier against contaminants.

C-Peptides of Proinsulin Test System A Class I device intended to measure C-peptides of proinsulin levels in serum, plasma, and urine. Measurements of C-peptides of proinsulin are used in the diagnosis and treatment of patients with abnormal insulin secretion, including diabetes mellitus.

C-Reactive Protein Immunological Test System A Class II device that consists of the reagents used to measure by immunochemical techniques the C-reactive protein in serum, plasma, and body fluids. Measurements of C-reactive protein aids in evaluation of the amount of injury to body tissues.

Calcitonin Test System A Class II device intended to measure the thyroid hormone calcitonin (thyrocalcitonin) levels in plasma and serum. Calcitonin measurements are used in the diagnosis and treatment of diseases involving the thyroid and parathyroid glands, including carcinoma and hyperparathyroidism (excessive activity of the parathyroid gland).

Calcium Hydroxide Cavity Liner A Class I device made of material that is applied to the interior of a prepare cavity and provides protection for the pulp of the tooth. The device is applied to the area to be restored prior to the insertion of restorative material, such as amalgam.

Calcium Test System A Class II device intended to measure the total calcium level in serum. Calcium measurements are used in the diagnosis and treatment of parathyroid disease, a variety of bone diseases, chronic renal disease and tetany (intermittent muscular contractions or spasms).

Calculator/Data Processing Module for Clinical Use An electronic Class I device intended to store, retrieve, and process laboratory data.

Calculus Removal, Hand-held Instrument A Class II hand-held metal scraper device used to remove calculus deposits from tooth surfaces.

Calibration Gas A Class II device consisting of a container of gas of known concentration used to calibrate gas concentration measurement devices.

Calibrator A Class II device intended for medical purposes for use in a test system to establish points of reference that are used in the determination of values in the measurement of substances in human specimens.

Calibrator for Cell Indices A Class III device that approximates whole blood or certain blood cells and that is used to set an instrument intended to measure mean cell volume (MCV), mean cell diameter (MCD), mean corpuscular hemoglobin (MCH), mean corpuscular hemoglobin concentration (MCHC), or other cell indices. It is a suspension of particles or fixed cells whose size, shape, concentration, and other characteristics have been carefully determined.

Calibrator for Hemoglobin and Hematocrit Measurement A Class II device that approximates whole blood, red blood cells, or a hemoglobin derivative and that is used to set instruments intended to measure hemoglobin, the hematocrit, or both. It is a material whose characteristics have been carefully determined.

Calibrator for Platelet Counting A Class III device that approximates platelets in plasma and that is used to set a platelet counting instrument. It is a suspension of particles or fixed cells whose size, particles or fixed cells whose size, shape, concentration, and other characteristics have been carefully determined.

Calipers for Clinical Use A compasslike Class I device intended for use in measuring the thickness or diameter of a part of the body or the distance between two body surfaces, such as for measuring an excised skeletal specimen to determine the proper replacement size of a prosthesis.

Cane A Class I device used to provide minimum weight support while walking. Examples of canes include the following: a standard cane, a forearm cane, and a cane with a tripod, quad, or retractable stud on the ground end.

Cane, Crutch, and Walker Tips Class I rubber accessories applied to the ground end of mobility aids to prevent skidding.

Cannabinoid Test System A Class II device intended to measure any of the cannabinoids, hallucinogenic compounds endogenous to marihuana, in serum, plasma, saliva, and urine. Cannabinoid compounds include δ-9-tetrahydrocannabinol cannabidiol, cannabinol, and cannabichromene. Measurements obtained by this device are used in the diagnosis and treatment of cannabinoid use or abuse and in monitoring levels of cannabinoids during clinical investigational use.

Capillary Blood Collection Tube A Class I, plain or heparinized glass tube of very small diameter used to collect blood by capillary action.

Carbon Dioxide Absorbent A Class II device consisting of an absorbent material (e.g., soda lime) used to remove carbon dioxide from the gases in a breathing circuit.

Carbon Dioxide Absorber A Class II device used in a breathing circuit as a container for the carbon dioxide absorbent. It may include a canister and water drain.

Carbon Dioxide Gas Analyzer A Class II diagnostic anesthesiology device, used to measure the concentration of carbon dioxide in a gas mixture as an aid in determining the patient's ventilatory, circulatory, and metabolic status. The device may use analytical techniques such as chemical titration, absorption of infrared radiation, gas chromatography, and mass spectrometry.

Carbon Monoxide Gas Analyzer A Class II diagnostic anesthesiology device, used to measure the concentration of carbon monoxide in a gas mixture as an aid in determining the patient's ventilatory, circulatory, and metabolic status. The device may use analytical techniques such as chemical titration, absorption of infrared radiation, gas chromatography, and mass spectrometry.

Carbon Monoxide Test System A Class I device intended to measure carbon monoxide or carboxy-hemoglobin (carbon monoxide bound to the hemoglobin in the blood) in blood. Measurements obtained by this device are used in the diagnosis and treatment of, or confirmation of, carbon monoxide poisoning.

Carbonic Anhydrase B and C Immunological Test System A Class I device that consists of the reagents used to measure, by immunochemical techniques, the specific carbonic anhydrase protein molecules in human serum and other body fluids. Measurements of carbonic anhydrase B and C aid in the diagnosis of abnormal hemoglobin metabolism.

Carboxyhemoglobin Assay A Class II device used to determine the carboxyhemoglobin (the compound formed when hemoglobin is exposed to carbon monoxide) content of human blood as an aid in the diagnosis of carbon monoxide poisoning. This measurement may be made using methods such as spectroscopy, colorimetry, spectrophotometry, and gasometry.

Carboxymethylcellulose Sodium 32% and Ethylene Oxide Homopolymer 13% Denture Adhesive A Class I device that is applied to the base of a denture before the denture is inserted into the patient's mouth. The device is used to improve denture retention and comfort.

Carboxymethylcellulose Sodium 40–100% Denture Adhesive A Class I device that is applied to the base of a denture before the denture is inserted into the patient's mouth. The device is used to improve denture retention and comfort.

Carboxymethylcellulose Sodium 13% and Ethylene Oxide Homopolymer Denture Adhesive A Class I device that is applied to the base of a denture before the denture is inserted into the patient's mouth. The device is used to improve denture retention and comfort.

Carboxymethylcellulose Sodium 49% and Ethylene Oxide Homopolymer 21% Denture Adhesive A Class I device that is applied to the base of a denture before the denture is inserted into the patient's mouth. The device is used to improve denture retention and comfort.

Carboxymethylcellulose Sodium and Cationic Polyacrylamide Polymer Denture Adhesive A Class I device that is applied to the base of a denture before the denture is inserted into the patient's mouth. The device is used to improve denture retention and comfort.

Cardiac Monitor (Including cardiotachometer and rate alarm) A Class II device device used to measure the heart rate from an analog signal produced by an electrocardiograph, vectorcardiograph, or blood pressure monitor. This device may sound an alarm when the heart rate falls outside present upper and lower limits.

Cardiac Pacemaker (External transcutaneous) A Class III device used to supply a periodic electrical impulse intended to pace the heart. The device is usually applied to the surface of the chest through electrodes such as defibrillator paddles.

Cardiopulmonary Bypass (CPB) A Class III multicomponent device designed to perform the dual function of the heart and lungs during open heart surgery.

Cardiopulmonary Bypass Accessory Equipment A Class II device that is equipment, which includes devices having no contact with blood-material, used in the cardiopulmonary bypass circuit to support, adjoin, or connect components or to aid in the setup of the extracorporeal line, e.g., an oxygenator mounting bracket or system priming equipment.

Cardiopulmonary Bypass Arterial Line Blood Filter A Class III device used as part of a gas exchange (oxygenator) system to filter nonbiologic articles and emboli out of the blood. It is used in the arterial return line.

Cardiopulmonary Bypass Blood Pump A Class II device that uses a revolving roller mechanism to pump blood through the circuit during open heart surgery.

Cardiopulmonary Bypass Blood Reservoir A Class II device used in conjunction with short-term, extracorporeal circulation devices to hold a reserve supply of blood in the bypass circulation. (If a reservoir contains a defoamer or filter, it is classified into the same category as the defoamer or filter.)

Cardiopulmonary Bypass Bubble Detector A Class II device used to detect bubbles in the arterial return line of the cardiopulmonary bypass circuit.

Cardiopulmonary Bypass Cardiotomy Return Sucker A Class II device consisting of tubing, a connector, and a probe or tip that is used to remove blood from the chest or heart during cardiopulmonary bypass surgery.

Cardiopulmonary Bypass Cardiotomy Suction Line Blood Filter A Class II device used as part of a gas exchange (oxygenator) system to filter biologic particles and emboli out of the blood. This device is intended for use in the cardiotomy suction line.

Cardiopulmonary Bypass Catheter, Cannula, and Tubing A Class II device, comprising catheters, cannulas, and tubing, used in cardiopulmonary bypass surgery to cannulate vessels, perfuse the coronary arteries, and interconnect with an oxygenator/perfusion pump apparatus.

Cardiopulmonary Bypass Coronary Pressure Gauge A Class II device used in cardiovascular bypass surgery to measure the pressure of the blood perfusing the coronary arteries.

Cardiopulmonary Bypass Defoamer A Class III device used in conjunction with an oxygenator during open heart surgery to remove gas bubbles from the pumped blood.

Cardiopulmonary Bypass Fitting, Manifold, Stopcock, and Adaptor Class II devices used in cardiovascular diagnostic, surgical, and therapeutic applications to interconnect tubing, catheters, and other devices.

Cardiopulmonary Bypass Gas Control Unit A Class II device used to control and measure the flow of gas into the oxygenator. The device is calibrated for a specific gas.

Cardiopulmonary Bypass Heat Exchanger A Class II device, consisting of a heat exchange system, to warm or cool the blood or perfusion fluid flowing through the device.

Cardiopulmonary Bypass In-Line Blood Gas Sensor A Class II device that is a transducer device that measures the level of gases in the blood.

Cardiopulmonary Bypass Intracardiac Suction Control A Class II device used to provide the vacuum and control for a cardiotomy return sucker.

Cardiopulmonary Bypass Level Sensing Monitor and/or Control A Class II device used to monitor and/or control the level of blood in the blood reservoir and to sound an alarm when the level falls below a predetermined value.

Cardiopulmonary Bypass Nonroller-Type Blood Pump A Class III device that uses a method other than revolving rollers to pump the blood through the cardiopulmonary bypass circuit during bypass surgery.

Cardiopulmonary Bypass On-Line Blood Gas Monitor   A Class II device used in conjunction with a blood sensor to measure the level of gases in the blood.

Cardiopulmonary Bypass Oxygenator   A Class III device used to exchange gases between blood and a gaseous environment to satisfy the gas exchange needs of a patient during open-heart surgery.

Cardiopulmonary Bypass Pulsatile Flow Generator   A Class III electrically and pneumatically operated device used to create pulsatile blood flow. The device is placed in a cardiopulmonary bypass circuit downstream from the oxygenator.

Cardiopulmonary Bypass Pump Speed Control   A Class II device that incorporates an electrical system, mechanical system, or both, and is used to control the speed of blood pumps used in cardiopulmonary bypass surgery.

Cardiopulmonary Bypass Pump Tubing   A Class II device composed of polymeric tubing used in the blood pump head that is cyclically compressed by the pump to cause the blood to flow through the cardiopulmonary bypass circuit.

Cardiopulmonary Bypass Roller-Type Blood Pump   A Class II device that uses a roller mechanism to pump the blood through the cardiopulmonary bypass circuit during bypass surgery.

Cardiopulmonary Bypass Temperature Controller   A Class II device used to control the temperature of the fluid entering and leaving a heat exchanger.

Cardiopulmonary Bypass Tubing   A Class II device, consisting of polymeric tubing that is used in the pump head, where it is cyclically compressed by the rotors to cause the blood to flow through the bypass circuit.

Cardiopulmonary Emergency Cart   A Class I device used to store and transport resuscitation supplies. The device is related to delivery of proper emergency treatment, but it does not include any equipment used in cardiopulmonary resuscitation.

Cardiopulmonary Prebypass Filter   A Class II device used during priming of the oxygenator circuit to remove particulates or other debris from the circuit prior to initiating bypass. The device is not to be used to filter blood.

Cardiovascular Blood Flowmeter   A Class II device connected to a flow transducer that energizes the transducer and processes and displays the blood flow signal.

Cardiovascular Flowmeter   A Class II device that, when connected to a flow transducer, energizes the transducer and displays the blood flow signal.

Cardiovascular Intravascular Filter A Class II implanted device placed in the inferior vena cava for the purpose of preventing pulmonary thromboemboli from flowing into the right side of the heart and into the pulmonary circulation.

Cardiovascular Surgical Instruments Class II devices that have special features for use in cardiovascular surgery. These devices include forceps, retractors, and scissors.

Carotid Sinus Nerve Stimulator A Class III device used to decrease arterial pressure by stimulating Hering's nerve at the carotid sinus.

Cartridge Syringe A Class I device used to inject anesthetic agents subcutaneously or intramuscularly. The device consists of a metal syringe body into which a disposable, previously filled, glass carpule (a cylindrical cartridge) containing anesthetic is placed. After attaching a needle to the syringe body and activating the carpule by partially inserting the plunger on the syringe, the device is used to administer an injection into the patient.

Cast Component A Class I device intended for medical purposes to protect or support a cast. This generic type of device includes the cast heel, toe cap, cast support, and walking iron.

Cast Removal Instrument An AC-powered, hand-held Class I device intended to remove a cast from a patient. This generic type of device includes the electric cast cutter and cast vacuum.

Catecholamines (Total) Test System A Class I device intended to determine whether a group of similar compounds (epinephrine, norepinephrine, and dopamine) are present in urine and plasma. Catecholamine determinations are used in the diagnosis and treatment of adrenal medulla and hypertensive disorders, and for catecholamine-secreting tumors (pheochromocytoma, neuroblastoma, ganglioneuroma, and retinoblastoma).

Catheter (Biliary, and accessories) A Class II tubular, flexible device used for temporary or prolonged drainage of the biliary tract, for splinting of the bile duct during healing, or for preventing stricture of the bile duct. This generic type of device may include a bile collecting bag that is attached to the biliary catheter by a connector and fastened to the patient with a strap.

Catheter (Continent ileostomy) A Class II flexible tubular device used as a form during surgery for continent ileostomy and it provides drainage after surgery. Additionally, the device may be inserted periodically by the patient for routine care to empty the ileal pouch. This generic type of device includes the rectal catheter for continent ileostomy.

Catheter (Continuous flush) A Class II device used as an attachment to a catheter-transducer system that permits continuous intravascular flushing at a slow infusion rate for the purpose of eliminating clotting, back-leakage, and waveform damping.

Catheter (Electrode recording and electrode probe) A Class II device, or devices, used to detect an intracardiac electrocardiogram, or to detect cardiac output or left-to-right heart shunts. The devices may be unipolar or multipolar for electrocardiogram detection, or may be a platinum-tipped catheter that senses the presence of a special indicator for cardiac output or left-to-right heart shunt determinations.

Catheter (Embolectomy) A Class II device that is a balloon-tipped catheter used to remove thromboemboli that have migrated from blood vessels from one site in the vascular tree to another.

Catheter (Fiberoptic oximeter) A Class II device used to estimate the oxygen saturation of the blood. It consists of two fiberoptic bundles that conduct light at a desired wavelength through blood and detect the reflected and scattered light at the distal end of the catheter.

Catheter (Flow-directed) A Class II device that incorporates a gas-filled balloon to help direct the catheter to the desired position.

Catheter (Nasopharyngeal catheter) A nasopharyngeal catheter is a Class II device consisting of a bougie or filiform catheter that is intended for use in probing or dilating the eustachian tube. This generic type of device includes eustachian catheters.

Catheter (Percutaneous) A Class II device that is introduced into a vein or artery through the skin using a dilator and a sheath or guide wire.

Catheter (Septostomy) A Class II device composed of a special balloon catheter that is used to create or enlarge the atrial septal defect found in the heart of infants.

Catheter (Steerable) A Class II device used for diagnostic and monitoring purposes whose movements are directed by a steering control unit.

Catheter (Steerable control system) A Class II device that is connected to the proximal end of a steerable guide wire that controls the motion of the steerable catheter.

Catheter Balloon Repair Kit A Class II device used to repair or replace the balloon of a balloon catheter. The kit contains the materials necessary to effect the repair or replacement, such as glue and new balloons.

Catheter Cannula A Class II device consisting of a hollow tube which is inserted into a vessel or cavity. This device provides a rigid or semirigid structure that can be connected to a tube or connector.

Catheter Guide Holder A Class I device that holds a spring guide during percutaneous techniques and during storage and sterilization.

Catheter Guide Wire A Class II device consisting of a coiled wire that is designed to fit inside a percutaneous catheter for the purpose of directing the catheter through a blood vessel.

Catheter Percutaneous Introducer A Class II device consisting of a sheath used to facilitate placing a catheter through the skin into a vein or artery.

Catheter Stylet A Class II device consisting of a wire that is run through a catheter or cannula to render it stiff.

Catheter Tip Occluder A Class II device that is inserted into certain catheters to prevent flow through one or more orifices.

Catheter Tip Pressure Transducer A Class II device incorporated into the distal end of a catheter. When placed in the bloodstream its mechanical or electrical properties change in relation to changes in blood pressure. These changes are in turn transmitted to accessory equipment for analysis.

Cavity Varnish A Class I device that consists of a compound used to coat a prepared cavity of a tooth prior to insertion of restorative materials, such as amalgam, into the dentinal tissue.

Cell Enzyme Assay A Class II device used to measure the activity in red cells, white cells, or both, of various clinically important enzymes and metabolites, such as pyruvate kinase and 2,3-diphosphoglycerate. A red cell enzyme assay is used to determine the enzyme defects responsible for a patient's hereditary hemolytic anemia.

Cell Freezing Apparatus and Reagents for in vitro Diagnostic Use Class I devices used to freeze human red blood cells for in vitro diagnostic use.

Cell and Tissue Culture Supplies and Equipment Class I devices that are used to examine, propagate, nourish, or grow cells and tissue cultures. These include such articles as slide culture chambers, perfusion and roller apparatus, cell culture suspension systems, and tissue culture flasks, disks, tubes, and roller bottles.

Cement Dispenser A nonpowered, syringe-like Class I device intended for use in placing bone cement into surgical sites.

Cement Mixer for Clinical Use A Class I device consisting of a container intended for use in mixing bone cement.

Cement Monomer Vapor Evacuator A Class I device intended for use during surgery to contain or remove undesirable fumes, such as monomer vapor from bone cement.

Cement Ventilation Tube A tube-like Class I device usually made of plastic intended to be inserted into a surgical cavity to allow the release of air or fluid from the cavity as it is being filled with bone cement.

Centrifugal Chemistry Analyzer for Clinical Use An automatic Class I device intended to centrifugally mix a sample and a reagent and spectrophotometrically measure concentrations of the sample constituents. This device is intended for use in conjunction with certain materials to measure a variety of analytes.

Cephalometer A Class II device used in dentistry during X-ray procedures. The device is used to place and to hold a patient's head in a standard position during dental X-ray.

Ceruloplasmin Immunological Test System A Class II device that consists of the reagents used to measure, by immunochemical techniques, the ceruloplasmin (copper-transporting serum protein) in serum, body fluids, or tissues. Measurements of ceruloplasmin aid in the diagnosis of copper metabolism disorders.

Cervical Cap A Class II device composed of a flexible, cup-like receptacle that fits over the cervix to collect menstrual flow or to aid artificial insemination. This generic type of device is not to be used as a contraceptive.

Cervical Drain A Class II device designed to provide an exit channel for draining discharge from the cervix after pelvic surgery.

Chamber (Patient care reverse isolation) A Class II device consisting of a room-like enclosure designed to prevent the entry of harmful airborne material. This device protects a patient who is undergoing treatment for burns or is lacking a normal immunosuppressive defense due to therapy or congenital abnormality. The device includes fans and air filters which maintain an atmosphere of clean air at a pressure greater than the air pressure outside the enclosure.

Chilling Unit A refrigerative Class II device used to chill and maintain cold packs at a reduced temperature.

Chin Prosthesis A Class II silicone rubber solid device intended to be implanted, to augment, or to reconstruct the chin.

***Chlamydia* Serological Reagents** Class I devices that consist of antigens and antisera used in serological tests to identify chlamydial antibodies in a patient's serum. Additionally, some of these reagents consist of chlamydia antisera conjugated with a fluorescent dye and are used to identify chlamydia directly from clinical specimens and/or cultured isolates derived from clinical specimens. The identification aids in the diagnosis of disease caused by bacteria belonging to the genus *Chlamydia* and provides epidemiological information on diseases caused by these microorganisms. Chlamydia are the causative agents of psittacosis (a form of pneumonia), lympho-granuloma venereum (a venereal disease), and trachoma (a chronic disease of the eye and eyelid).

Chloride Test System   A Class II device intended to measure the level of chloride in plasma, serum, sweat, and urine. Chloride measurements are used in the diagnosis and treatment of electrolyte and metabolic disorders, such as cystic fibrosis and diabetic acidosis.

Cholesterol (Total) Test System   A Class I device intended to measure cholesterol in plasma and serum. Cholesterol measurements are used in the diagnosis and treatment of disorders involving excess cholesterol in the blood and lipid and lipoprotein metabolism disorders.

Cholinesterase Test System   A Class I device intended to measure cholinesterase (an enzyme that catalyzes the hydrolysis of acetyl-choline to choline) in human specimens. There are two principal types of cholinesterase in human tissues. True cholinesterase is present at nerve endings and in erythrocytes (red blood cells) but is not present in plasma. Pseudo cholinesterase is present in plasma and liver but is not present in erythrocytes. Measurements obtained by this device are used in the diagnosis and treatment of cholines-terase inhibition disorders (e.g., insecticide poisoning and suc-cinylcholine poisoning).

Cholylglycine Test System   A Class II device intended to measure the bile acid cholylglycine in serum. Measurements obtained by this device are used in the diagnosis and treatment of liver disorders, such as cirrhosis or obstructive liver disease.

Chromatographic Separation Material for Clinical Use   A Class I device accessory (e.g., ion exchange absorbents, ion exchange resins, and ion papers) intended for use in ion exchange chroma-tography, a procedure in which a compound is separated from a solution.

Chromosome Culture Kit   A Class I device containing the necessary ingredients (e.g., Minimum Essential Media (MEM) or McCoy's 5A culture media, phytohemagglutinin, fetal calf serum, antibiotics, and heparin) used to culture tissues for diagnosis of congenital chromosome abnormalities.

Chronaximeter   A Class II device that measures neuromuscular ex-citability by means of a strength-duration curve that provides a basis for diagnosis and prognosis of neurological dysfunction.

Chymotrypsin Test System   A Class I device intended to measure the activity of the enzyme chymotrypsin in blood and other body fluids and in feces. Chymotrypsin measurements are used in the diagnosis and treatment of pancreatic exocrine insufficiency.

35

Cine or Spot Fluorographic X-ray Camera A Class II device intended to photograph diagnostic images produced by X-rays with an image intensifier.

Circumcision Instrument A Class II device made specifically for use in circumcision procedures. This generic type of device includes the plastic bell circumcision device, circumcision shield, and circumcision clamp.

***Citrobaxter* spp. Serological Reagents** A Class I device that consists of antigen and antisera used in serological tests to identify *Citrobaxter* spp. from cultured isolates derived from clinical specimens. The identification aids in the diagnosis of disease caused by bacteria belonging to the genus *Citrobaxter* and provides epidemiological information on diseases caused by these microorganisms. *Citrobaxter* spp. have occasionally been associated with urinary tract infections.

Class I Devices, General Controls Primarily intended for devices that pose no potential risk to health, and thus can be adequately regulated without imposing standards or the need for premarket review. This category provides a broad general control. It requires that manufacturers of these devices register with the FDA, provide a listing of products, maintain adequate reports, and comply with good manufacturing practices. Examples: stethoscope, periodontic syringes, nebulizers, and vaginal insufflators.

Class II Devices, Performance Standards Applicable when general controls are not adequate to assure the safety and effectiveness of a device based on the potential risk to health posed by the device. To classify a device in the Class II category, the FDA must find that enough data are available on which to base adequate performance standards that would control the safety and effectiveness of these devices. Examples: diagnostic catheters, electrocardiographs, wound dressings, percutaneous catheters, and gastrointestinal irrigation systems.

Class III Devices, Premarket Approval Applicable when a device is a "critical device," i.e., life-supporting and/or life-sustaining, unless adequate justification is given for classifying it in another category. Class III contains devices produced after 1976 that are not sufficiently similar to pre-1976 devices, and devices that were regulated as new drugs before 1976. Examples: bronchial tubes, ventilators, vascular grafts, pacemakers, cardiopulmonary bypass, and surgical meshes.

Cleaner (Recirculating air) A Class II device used to remove particles from the air by electrostatic precipitation or filtration.

Clinical Color Change Thermometer A Class II device used to measure oral or rectal body temperature by displaying the color changes of heat sensitive liquid crystals. It is a disposable device with the liquid crystals (cholesteric esters) sealed in plastic at the end of a plastic strip.

Clinical Electronic Thermometer A Class II device used to measure the body temperature of a patient by means of a transducer coupled with an electronic signal amplification, conditioning, and display unit. The transducer may be in a detachable probe with or without a disposable cover.

Clinical Mercury Thermometer A Class II device used to measure oral, rectal, or axillary body temperature using the thermal expansion of mercury.

Clinical Sample Concentrator A Class I device intended to concentrate (by dialysis, evaporation, etc.) serum, urine, cerebrospinal fluid, and other body fluids before the fluids are analyzed.

Clinical Toxicology Calibrator A Class II device intended for medical purposes for use in a test system to establish points of reference that are used in the determination of values in the measurement of substances in human specimens. A clinical toxicology calibrator can be a mixture of drugs or a specific material for a particular drug (e.g., ethanol, lidocaine, etc.).

Clinical Toxicology Control Material A Class I device intended to provide an estimation of the precision of a device test system and to detect and monitor systematic deviations from accuracy resulting from reagent or instrument defects. This generic type of device includes various single, and multianalyte control materials.

Clip (Implantable clip) A clip-like Class II device intended to connect internal tissues to aid healing. It is not absorbable.

Clip (Removable skin clip) A clip-like Class I device intended to connect skin tissues temporarily to aid healing. It is not absorbable.

Clip (Vascular) A Class II implanted device designed to occlude, by compression, blood flow in small blood vessels.

Clip (Vena cava) A Class II implanted device designed to partially occlude the vena cava for the purpose of inhibiting the flow of thromboemboli through that vessel.

Closed-Circuit Television Reading System A Class I device that consists of a lens, video camera, and video monitor that is intended for use by a patient who has subnormal vision to magnify reading material.

Coagulase Plasma A Class II device that consists of freeze-dried animal or human plasma that is used for performance of coagulase tests primarily on staphylococcal bacteria. When reconstituted, the fluid plasma is clotted by the action of the enzyme coagulase which is produced by pathogenic staphylococci. Test results are used primarily as an aid in the diagnosis of disease caused by pathogenic bacteria belonging to the genus *Staphylococcus* and provide epidemiological information on diseases caused by these microorganisms. The chief sources of a staphylococcal infection are accessible human lesions, the respiratory tract, and the skin. Staphylococci can survive for a period of time outside the body in the air. The airborne infection potential is important in hospitals because a large proportion of the staff and patients carry antibiotic resistant staphylococci in the nose, the throat, or on the skin. Introduction of large quantities of airborne pathogenic staphylococci bacterid into newborn nurseries and surgical operating rooms may lead to serious clinical disease (e.g., abscesses in the organs). The coagulase test is a key test for differentiating the pathogenic (coagulase producing) strains of staphylococcal bacteria from the nonpathogenic strains. The literature review disclosed appreciable lot-to-lot variations in the purity and stability of coagulase plasmas which often lead to problems of false-positive and false-negative test results. The source of supply of coagulase plasma appears to be a factor in the occurrence of a false-positive test result. The coagulation in the test tube seems to involve the conversion of fibrinogen to fibrin by the coagulase enzyme complex and the coagulase-reacting factor in the plasma.

Coagulation Instrument An automated or semiautomated Class II device used to determine the onset of clot formation for in vitro coagulation studies.

Coating Material for Rein Fillings A Class I device that is applied to the surface of a restorative resin dental filling in order to attain a smooth, glaze-like finish on the surface of the filling.

Cobalt Chrome Molybdenum Subperiosteal Implant Material A Class II device used to construct custom prosthetic devices which are surgically implanted into the lower or upper jaw between the periosteum (connective tissue covering the bone) and supporting bony structures. The device provides support for prostheses, such as dentures.

Cocaine and Cocaine Metabolite Test System A Class II device intended to measure cocaine and a cocaine metabolite (benzoylecgonine) in serum, plasma, and urine. Measurements obtained by this device are used in the diagnosis and treatment of cocaine use or overdose.

***Coccidioides immitis* Serological Reagents** Class II devices that consist of antigens and antisera used in serological tests to identify *Coccidioides immitis* antibodies in a patient's serum. The identification aids in the diagnosis of coccidioidomycosis caused by a fungus belonging to the genus *Coccidioides* and provide epidemiological information on diseases caused by this microorganism. An infection with *Coccidioides immitis* produces symptoms varying in severity from those accompanying the common cold to those of influenza.

Codeine Test System   A Class II device intended to measure codeine (a narcotic, pain-relieving drug) in serum and urine. Measurements obtained by this device are used in the diagnosis and treatment of codeine use or overdose, and in monitoring levels of codeine to ensure appropriate therapy.

Cohn Fraction II Immunological Test System   A Class I device that consists of reagents that contain, or are used to measure, that fraction of plasma containing protein gamma globulins, predominately of the IgG class. The device may be used as coprecipitant in radio-immunoassay methods, as raw material for the purification of IgG subclasses, and to reduce nonspecific adsorption of plasma proteins in immunoassay techniques. Measurement of these proteins aids in the diagnosis of any disease concerned with abnormal levels of IgG gamma globulins, such as agammaglobulinemia or multiple myeloma.

Cohn Fraction IV Immunological Test System (2243)   A Class I device that consists of, or measures, that fraction of plasma proteins, predominantly α- and β-globulins, used as a raw material for the production of pure α- or β-globulins. Measurement of specific α- or β-globulins aids in the diagnosis of many diseases, such as Wilson's disease (an inherited disease affecting the liver and brain), Tangier's disease (absence of α-lipoprotein), malnutrition, iron deficiency anemia, red blood cell disorders, and kidney disease.

Cohn Fraction V Immunological Test System   A Class I device that consists of, or measures, that fraction of plasma containing predominately albumin (a plasma protein). This test aids in the diagnosis of diseases where albumin levels may be depressed, e.g., nephrosis (disease of the kidney), proteinuria (protein in the urine), gastroenteropathy (disease of the stomach and small intestine), rheumatoid arthritis, and viral hepatitis.

Cold Pack   A Class I device consisting of a compact fabric envelope containing a specially hydrated (chemically combined with water) pliable silicate gel capable of forming to the contour of the body. It is used when cold therapy is indicated for body surfaces.

Colduscope and Accessories   A Class II device designed to permit direct viewing of the organs within the peritoneum by a telescopic system introduced into the pelvic cavity through the posterior vaginal fornix. It is used to perform diagnostic and surgical procedures on the female genital organs. This generic type of device may include: trocar and cannula, instruments used through an operating channel, scope preheaters, light source and cables, and component parts.

Colonic Irrigation System A Class II device intended to instill water into the colon through a nozzle inserted into the rectum to cleanse (evacuate) the contents of the lower colon. The system is designed to allow evacuation of the colonic contents during administration of the nozzle via tubing and includes a system which enables the pressure, temperature, or water flow through the nozzle to be controlled. The device may include a console-type toilet and necessary fittings to allow the device to be connected to water and sewer pipes. The device may use electrical power to heat the water.

Color Vision Plate Illuminator An AC-powered Class I device that is a lamp intended to illuminate properly color vision testing plates. It may include a filter.

Color Vision Tester A Class I device that consists of various colored materials, such as colored yarns or color vision plates (multicolored plates which patients with color vision deficiency would perceive as being of one color), intended to evaluate color vision.

Colorimeter, Photometer, or Spectrophotometer for Clinical Use A Class I instrument intended to measure radiant energy emitted, transmitted, absorbed, or reflected under controlled conditions. This device may include a monochromator to produce light of a specific wavelength.

Colostomy Rod A Class II device used during the loop colostomy procedure. A loop of colon is surgically brought out through the abdominal wall and the stiff colostomy rod is placed through the loop temporarily to keep the colon from slipping back through the surgical opening.

Colostrum Immunological Test System A Class I device that consists of the reagents used to measure by immunochemical techniques the specific proteins in colostrum. Colostrum is a substance excreted by the mammary glands during pregnancy and until production of breast milk begins one to five days after childbirth.

Colposcope A Class II device designed to permit direct viewing of the tissues of the vagina and cervix by a telescopic system located outside the vagina. It is used to diagnose abnormalities and select an area for biopsy. This generic type of device may include a light source, cables, and component parts.

Complement C, Inhibitor (Inactivator) Immunological Test System A Class II device that consists of the reagents used to measure, by immunochemical techniques, the complement C1 inhibitor (a plasma protein) in serum. The complement C1 inhibitor occurs normally in plasma and blocks the action of the C1 component of complement (a group of serum proteins that destroy infectious agents). Measurement of complement C1 inhibitor aids in the diagnosis of hereditary angioneurotic edema (increased blood vessel permeability causing swelling of tissues) and a rare form of angioedema associated with lymphoma (lymph node cancer).

Complement C3₆ Inactivator Immunological Test System A Class II device that consists of the reagents used to measure, by immunochemical techniques, the complement $C3_b$ inactivator (a plasma protein in serum). Complement is a group of serum proteins that destroy infectious agents. Measurement of complement $C3_b$ inactivator aids in the diagnosis of inherited antibody dysfunction.

Complement Components Immunological Test System A Class II device that consists of the reagents used to measure, by immunochemical techniques, complement components C1q, C1r, C1s, C2, C3, C4, C5, C6, C7, C8, and C9 in serum biological fluids, and tissues. Complement C1s is a group of serum proteins that destroy infectious agents. Measurement of these proteins aid in the diagnosis of immunologic disorders, especially deficiencies of complement components.

Complement Reagents A Class I device that consists of naturally occurring serum protein from any warm-blooded animal (such as guinea pigs) that may be included as a component part of serological test kits used in the diagnosis of disease.

Component Any material, substance, piece, part, or assembly used during device manufacture that is intended to be included in the finished device.

Compound S (11-Deoxycortisol) Test System A Class I device intended to measure the level of compound S (11-deoxycortisol) in plasma. Compound S is a steroid intermediate in the biosynthesis of the adrenal hormone cortisol. Measurements of compound S are used in the diagnosis and treatment of certain adrenal and pituitary gland disorders resulting in clinical symptoms of masculinization and hypertension.

Compressible Limb Sleeve A Class II device used to prevent pooling of blood in a limb by inflating periodically a sleeve around the limb.

Computed Tomography X-ray System A Class II diagnostic X-ray system intended to produce cross-sectional images of the body by computer reconstruction of X-ray transmission data from the same axial plane taken at different angles. This generic type of device may include signal analysis and display equipment, patient and equipment supports, component parts, and accessories.

Condom A Class II device composed of a sheath that completely covers the penis with a closely fitting membrane. The condom is used for contraception and for the prophylactic purpose of preventing transmission of venereal disease. The device may also be used to collect seminal fluid to aid in the diagnosis of infertility.

Congenital Hip Dislocation Abduction Splint   A Class I device used to stabilize the hips of a young child with dislocated hips in an abducted position (away from the midline).

Conjugated Sulfolithocholic Acid (SLCG) Test System   A Class II device intended to measure the bile acid SLCG in serum. Measurements obtained by this device are used in the diagnosis and treatment of liver disorders, such as cirrhosis or obstructive liver disease.

Contact Lens Heat Disinfection Unit   A Class III device intended to disinfect a contact lens by means of heat.

Contact Lens Inserter/Remover   A hand-held Class I device intended to insert or remove contact lenses by surface adhesion or suction.

Container   An I.V. container is a sterile Class II device for a fluid mixture to be administered to a patient.

Container for Collection and Processing of Blood and Blood Components   A Class I device composed of an empty plastic bag or plastic or glass bottle used to collect, store, or transfer blood and blood components for further processing.

Continent Ileostomy Catheter   A Class II flexible tubular device used as a form during surgery for continent ileostomy. It provides drainage after surgery. Additionally, the device may be inserted periodically by the patient for routine care to empty the ileal pouch. This generic type of device includes the rectal catheter for continent ileostomy.

Continuous Flow Sequential Multiple Chemistry Analyzer for Clinical Use   A Class I device that is a modular analytical instrument intended to simultaneously perform multiple chemical procedures using the principles of automated continuous flow systems. This device is intended for use in conjunction with certain materials to measure a variety of analytes.

Continuous Flush Catheter   A Class II device used as an attachment to a catheter-transducer system that permits continuous intravascular flushing at a slow infusion rate for the purpose of eliminating clotting, back-leakage, and waveform damping.

Contraceptive Diaphragm and Accessories   A Class II device consisting of a closely fitting membrane placed between the posterior aspect of the pubic bone and the posterior vaginal fornix. The device covers the cervix completely and is used to prevent pregnancy. The generic type of device may include an introducer and other accessories. Included in this generic type of device are those devices identified as: "contraceptive diaphragm" and "contraceptive diaphragm introducer."

Contraceptive Intrauterine Device (IUD) and Introducer   A Class III device placed high in the uterine fundus with a string extending from the uterus into the vagina and is used to prevent pregnancy. This generic type of device does not include products that function by drug activity, which are subject to the new drug provisions of the Federal Food, Drug, and Cosmetic Act.

Contraceptive Tubal Occlusion Device (TOD) and Introducer. A Class III device designed to close the fallopian tubes with a mechanical structure, e.g., a band or clip on the outside of the fallopian tubes or a plug or valve on the inside, that is used to prevent pregnancy. Included in this generic type of device are those devices identified as: "tubal occlusion band," "tubal occlusion clip," "tubal occlusion insert," and "tubal occlusion valve."

Control Number   Any distinctive combination of letters, numbers, or both, from which the complete manufacturing history, control, packaging and distribution of a production run, lot, or batch of finished devices can be determined.

Copper Sulfate Solution for Specific Gravity Determinations   A Class I device used to determine whether the hemoglobin content of a potential donor's blood meets the required level 12.5 grams per 100 milliliters of blood for women and 13.5 grams per 100 milliliters of blood for men.

Copper Test System   A Class I device intended to measure copper levels in plasma, serum, and urine. Measurements of copper are used in the diagnosis and treatment of anemia, infections, inflammations, and Wilson's disease (a hereditary disease primarily of the liver and nervous system). Test results are also used in monitoring patients with Hodgkin's disease (a disease primarily of the lymph system).

Corneal Electrode   An AC-powered Class II device, usually part of a special contact lens, intended to be applied directly to the cornea to provide data showing the changes in electrical potential in the retina after electroretinography (stimulation by light).

Corneal Radius Measuring Device   A Class I AC-powered device intended to measure corneal size by superimposing the image of the cornea on a scale at the focal length of the lens of a small, hand-held, single tube penscope or eye gauge magnifier.

Corticoids Test System   A Class I device intended to measure the levels of corticoids (hormones of the adrenal cortex) in serum and plasma. Measurements of corticoids are used in the diagnosis and treatment of disorders of the cortex of the adrenal glands, especially those associated with hypertension and electrolyte disturbances.

Corticosterone Test System   A Class I device intended to measure corticosterone (a steroid secreted by the adrenal gland) levels in plasma. Measurements of corticosterone are used in the diagnosis and treatment of adrenal disorders, such as adrenal cortex disorders and blocks in cortisol synthesis.

Cortisol (Hydrocortisone and hydroxycorticosterone) Test System A Class II device intended to measure the cortisol hormones secreted by the adrenal gland in plasma and urine. Measurements of cortisol are used in the diagnosis and treatment of disorders of the adrenal gland.

Corynebacterium **spp. Serological Reagents** Class I devices that consist of antisera conjugated with a fluorescent dye used to identify Corynebacterium spp. from clinical specimens. The identification aids in the diagnosis of disease caused by bacteria belonging to the genus *Corynebacterium* and provides epidemiological information on diseases caused by these microorganisms. The principal human pathogen of this genus, *Corynebacterium diphtheriae*, causes diphtheria. However, many other types of corynebacteria form part of the normal flora of the human respiratory tract, other mucus membranes, and skin, and are either nonpathogenic or have an uncertain pathogenic role.

Cotton Roll A Class I tube-shaped device composed of cotton fibers that is used to absorb moisture in the oral cavity during dental procedures.

Coxsackievirus Serological Reagents Class I devices that consist of antigens and antisera used in serological tests to identify coxsackievirus antibodies in a patient's serum. Additionally, some of these reagents consist of coxsackievirus antisera conjugated with a fluorescent dye that are used to identify coxsackievirus from clinical specimens and/or from tissue culture isolates derived from clinical specimens. The identification aids in the diagnosis of coxsackievirus infections and provides epidemiological information on diseases caused by these viruses. Coxsackieviruses produce a vareity of infections, including common colds, meningitis (inflammation of brain and spinal cord membranes), herpangina (brief fever accompanied by ulcerated lesions of the throat), and myopericarditis (inflammation of heart tissue).

Creatine Phosphokinase/Creatine Kinase or Isoenzymes Test System A Class II device intended to measure the activity of the enzyme creatine phosphokinase or its isoenzymes (a group of enzymes with similar biological activity) in plasma and serum. Measurements of creatine phosphokinase and its isoenzymes are used in the diagnosis and treatment of myocardial infarction and muscle diseases such as progressive, Duchenne-type muscular dystrophy.

Creatine Test System A Class I device intended to measure creatine (a substance synthesized in the liver and pancreas and found in biological fluids) in plasma, serum, and urine. Measurements of creatine are used in the diagnosis and treatment of muscle diseases;

endocrine disorders, including hyperthyroidism; in monitoring renal dialysis, and as a calculation basis for measuring other urine analytes.

Critical Component Any component of a critical device whose failure to perform can be reasonably expected to cause failure of a critical device, or to affect its safety or effectiveness.

Critical Device A device intended for surgical implant into the body or to support or sustain life, and whose failure to perform, when properly used in accordance with instructions for use provided in the labelling, can reasonably be expected to result in a significant injury to the user.

Critical Operation Any operation in the manufacture of a critical device that, if improperly performed, can be reasonably expected to cause the failure of a critical device or to affect its safety or effectiveness.

Crutch A Class I device used by disabled persons to provide minimal to moderate weight support while walking.

Cryophthalmic Unit A Class II device that is a probe with a small tip that becomes extremely cold through the controlled use of a refrigerant or gas. The device is intended to remove cataracts by the formation of an adherent ice ball in the lens, to freeze the eye and adjunct parts for surgical removal of scars, and to freeze tumors.

Cryosurgical Unit and Accessories (1) Cryosurgical unit with a liquid nitrogen cooled cryoprobe and accessories. A cryosurgical unit with a liquid nitrogen cooled cryoprobe and accessories is a Class II device intended to destroy tissue during surgical procedures by applying extreme cold. (2) Cryosurgical unit with a nitrous oxide cooled cryoprobe and accessories. A cryosurgical unit with a nitrous oxide cooled cryoprobe and accessories is a Class II device intended to destroy tissue during surgical procedures, including urological applications, by applying extreme cold. (3) Cryosurgical unit with a carbon dioxide cooled cryoprobe or a carbon dioxide dry ice applicator and accessories. A cryosurgical unit with a carbon dioxide cooled cryoprobe or a carbon dioxide dry ice applicator and accessories is a Class II device intended to destroy tissue during surgical procedures by applying extreme cold. The device is intended to treat disease conditions such as tumors, skin cancers, acne, scars, hemangiomas (benign tumors consisting of newly formed blood vessels), and various benign or malignant gynecological conditions affecting vulvar, vaginal, or cervical tissue. The device is not intended for urological applications.

***Cryptococcus neoformans* Serological Reagents** Class II devices that consist of antigens and antisera used in serological tests to identify *Cryptococcus neoformans* antibodies in a patient's serum. Additionally, some of these reagents consist of antisera conjugated

45

with a fluorescent dye (immunofluorescent reagents) and are used to identify *Cryptococcus neoformans* directly from clinical specimens and/or from cultured isolates derived from clinical specimens. The identification aids in the diagnosis of Cryptococcosis and provides epidemiological information on this type of disease. Cryptococcosis infections are found most often as chronic meningitis (inflammation of brain membranes) and, if not treated, are usually fatal.

Cuff Spreader   A Class I device used to install tracheal tube cuffs on tracheal and tracheotomy tubes.

Culture Medium for Antimicrobial Susceptibility Test   A Class II device that consists of any medium capable of supporting the growth of the majority of bacterial pathogens that require antimicrobial susceptibility tests. The medium is free of components known to be antagonistic to the common agents for which susceptibility tests are performed in the treatment of disease.

Culture Medium for Pathogenic *Neisseria* spp.   A Class II device that consists primarily of liquid and/or solid biological materials used to cultivate and identify pathogenic *Neisseria* spp. The identification aids in the diagnosis of disease caused by bacteria belonging to the genus *Neisseria* such as epidemic cerebrospinal meningitis, other meningococcal disease, and gonorrhea, and also provides epidemiological information on these diseases.

Cultured Animal and Human Cells   Class I in vitro cultivated cell lines from the tissue of humans or other animals that are used in various diagnostic procedures, particularly diagnostic virology and cytogenetic studies.

Cyclic AMP Test System   A Class II device intended to measure the level of adenosine 3,5-monophosphate (cyclic AMP) in plasma, urine, and other body fluids. Cyclic AMP measurements are used in the diagnosis and treatment of endocrine disorders, including hyperparathyroidism (overactivity of the parathyroid gland). Cyclic AMP measurements may also be used in the diagnosis and treatment of Graves' disease (a disorder of the thyroid) and in the differentiation of causes of hypercalcemia (elevated levels of serum calcium).

Cystine Test System   A Class I device intended to measure the amino acid cystine in urine. Cystine measurements are used in the diagnosis of cystinuria (occurrence of cystine in urine). Patients with cystinuria frequently develop kidney calculi (stones).

Cytocentrifuge   A Class I device used to concentrate cells from biological cell suspensions (e.g., cerebrospinal fluid) and to deposit these cells on a glass microscope slide for cytological examination.

Cytomegalovirus Serological Reagents   Class I devices that consist of antigens and antisera used in serological tests to identify cytomegalovirus antibodies in a patient's serum. The identification aids in the diagnosis of diseases caused by cytomegaloviruses (principally cytomegalic inclusion disease) and provides epidemiological information on these diseases. Cytomegalic inclusion disease is a generalized infection of infants and is caused by intrauterine or early postnatal infection with the virus. The disease may cause severe congenital abnormalities, such as microcephaly (abnormal smallness of the head), motor disability, and mental retardation. Cytomegalovirus infection has also been associated with acquired hemolytic anemia, acute and chronic hepatitis, and an infectious mononucleosis-like syndrome.

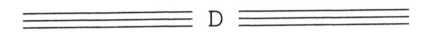

D

Daily Activity Assist Device   Class I devices that are modified adaptors and utensils (e.g., dressing, grooming, recreational activity, transfer, eating and homemaking aids) that are used to assist a patient in performing a specific function.

Defibrillator (DC)   A Class III device used to produce an electrical shock for defibrillating (restoring normal sinus rhythm) the atria or ventricles of the heart or to terminate other cardiac arrhythmias. The device may either synchronize the shock with the proper phase of the electrocardiogram or may operate asynchronously. The device delivers an electrical shock through paddles either directly across the heart or on the surface of the body.

Defibrillator Tester   A Class II device that is connected to the output of the defibrillator and is used to measure the energy delivered by the defibrillator into a standard resistive load. Some testers also provide waveform information.

Dehydroepiandoriterone (Free and Sulfate) Test System   A Class I device intended to measure dehydroepiandrosterone (DHEA) and its sulfate in urine, serum, plasma, and amniotic fluid. Dehydroepiandrosterone measurements are used in the diagnosis and treatment of DHEA-secreting adrenal carcinomas.

Denis Brown Splint   A Class I device used to immobilize the feet. It is used on young children with tibial torsion (excessive rotation of the lower leg) or club foot.

Densitometer   A Class II device used to measure the transmission of light through an indicator in a sample of blood.

Densitometer/Scanner (Integrating, reflectance, TLC, or radiochromatogram) for Clinical Use   A Class I device intended to measure the concentration of a substance on the surface of a film or other support media by either a photocell measurement of the light transmission through a given area of the medium, or, in the case of the radiochromatogram scanner, by measurement of the distribution of a specific radioactive element on a radiochromatogram.

Dental Amalgam Capsule   A Class I device that is a container in which silver alloy is mixed with mercury to form dental amalgam.

Dental Burr   A Class II rotary cutting device made from carbon steel or tungsten carbide used to cut hard mouth tissue, such as teeth or bone. It is also used to cut hard metals, plastics, porcelains, and similar materials that are used in the fabrication of dental devices.

Dental Cement   A Class II device used to affix dental filling materials and dental devices, such as crowns and bridges; to provide a restorative base for the protection of tooth pulp and to serve as temporary filling material for caries. The device is composed of materials such as zinc oxide-eugenol.

Dental Chair with Operative Unit   A Class I device that consists of an AC-powered chair or lounger in which the patient is positioned during dental procedures. Attached to the chair is an AC-powered operative unit that supplies power to, and serves as the base for, dental handpieces, lights, and other devices. It also holds syringes for air and water.

Dental Chair without Operative Unit   A Class I device that consists of an AC-powered chair or lounger in which the patient is positioned during dental procedures. The chair does not have an operative unit device attached.

Dental Depth Gauge Instrument   A Class I device consisting of a slender metal piece that is used in endodontic (root canal) treatment to prepare for placement of retentive or splinting pin. The device is used to measure the depth of a small hole in a tooth.

Dental Diamond Instrument   A Class II abrasive device used to smooth tooth surfaces during the fitting of crowns or bridges. The device consists of a shaft that is inserted into a handpiece and a head that has diamond chips imbedded in it. Rotation of the diamond instrument provides an abrasive action when it contacts the tooth.

Dental Electrosurgical Unit and Accessories   A Class II AC-powered device consisting of a controlled power source and a set of cutting and coagulating electrodes. This device is used to cut or remove soft tissue or to control bleeding during surgical procedures in the oral cavity. An electrical current passes through the tip of the electrode into the tissue and, depending upon the operating mode selected, cuts through soft tissue or coagulates the tissue.

Dental Floss A Class I string-like device made of cotton or other fibers that is intended to remove plaque and food particles from between the teeth to reduce tooth decay. The fibers of the device may be coated with wax for easier use.

Dental Hand Instrument A Class I hand-held device used to perform various tasks in general dentistry and oral surgery procedures. The following devices are included in this generic type of device: operative burnisher, operative amalgam carver, surgical bone chisel, operative amalgam and foil condenser, edodontic curette, operative currette, dental surgical elevator, operative dental excavator, operative explorer, surgical bone file, operative margin finishing file, periodontic file, periodontic probe, surgical rongeur forceps, surgical tooth extractor instrument, operative cutting instrument, operative matrix contouring instrument, operative margin-finishing knife, periodontic knife, periodontic marker, operative pliers, endodontic root-canal pulp-canal reamer, crown remover, periodontic scaler, collar and crown scissors, edondontic pulp-canal filling material spreader, and surgical osteotome chisel.

Dental Handle Instrument A Class I device made of metal or plastic that is used as a grip for working tips and mirrors used during dental procedures.

Dental Injecting Needle A Class II slender, hollow metal device with a sharp point that is attached to a syringe and is used to inject local anesthetics and other drugs.

Dental Matrix Band A Class I device made of stainless steel that is used as a mold and is placed around a tooth to provide support for restorative materials while filling a tooth.

Dental Mercury A Class II device composed of mercury that is used as a component in an amalgam alloy in the restoration of dental cavities or broken teeth.

Dental Operating Light A Class II AC-powered device used to illuminate oral structures and operating areas.

Dental Operative Unit A Class I AC-powered device that supplies power to, and serves as a base for, dental handpieces, lights or other dental devices and holds syringes for air and water. It can be attached to the dental chair or cabinets or located on a portable cart.

Dental Protector A Class II device used to protect the patient's teeth during intubation or other manipulative procedures within the oral cavity.

Dental Retractor A Class I device used to fold back oral tissues by pulling back the cheeks at the lips to aid operating procedures.

Dental Retractor Accessories A Class I device, such as a spring, that is used with a dental retractor (a device used to fold back oral tissue during operating procedures) to aid in pulling back the cheek as far as possible.

Dental X-ray Exposure Alignment Device A Class II device used to position and hold X-ray film, and to align the examination site with the X-ray beam.

Dental X-ray Film Holder A Class I device used to position and to hold X-ray film inside the mouth.

Dental X-ray Position Indicating Device A Class II device that is a collimator, cone, or aperture, that is used in dental radiographic examination. The device aligns the examination site with the X-ray beam and also restricts the dimensions of the dental X-ray field by limiting the size of the primary X-ray beam.

Denture Adhesive (Acacia, karaya gum and sodium borate) A Class III device that is applied to the base of a denture before the denture is inserted into the patient's mouth. The device is used to improve denture retention and comfort. There is a lack of information concerning the safety of adhesives containing sodium borate. Sodium borate concentration of 12–20% of the adhesive's total weight is equivalent to 2.6–5.3% boron. Because at least a portion of a dental adhesive is ingested, this amount of boron could cause chronic toxicity in denture wearers.

Denture Adhesive (Carboxymethylcellulose sodium and cationic polyacrylamide polymer) A Class I device that is applied to the base of a denture before the denture is inserted into the patient's mouth. The device is used to improve denture retention and comfort.

Denture Adhesive (Carboxymethylcellulose sodium 32% and ethylene oxide homopolymer 13%) A Class I device that is applied to the base of a denture before the denture is inserted into the patient's mouth. The device is used to improve denture retention and comfort.

Denture Adhesive (Carboxymethylcellulose sodium 40–100%) A Class I device that is applied to the base of a denture before the denture is inserted into the patient's mouth. The device is used to improve denture retention and comfort.

Denture Adhesive (Carboxymethylcellulose sodium 49% and ethylene oxide homopolymer 21%) A Class I device that is applied to the base of a denture before the denture is inserted into the patient's mouth. The device is used to improve denture retention and comfort.

Denture Adhesive (Karaya) A Class I device composed of karaya gum (a gum from the bark of a tree from the genus *Astragalus*) that is applied to the base of a denture before the denture is inserted into the patient's mouth. The device is used to improve denture retention and comfort.

Denture Adhesive (Karaya gum and ethylene oxide) A Class I device that is applied to the base of a denture before the denture is inserted into the patient's mouth. The device is used to improve denture retention and comfort.

Denture Adhesive (Karaya gum with sodium borate) A Class III device that is applied to the base of a denture before the denture is inserted into the patient's mouth. The device is used to improve denture retention and comfort. There is a lack of information concerning the safety of adhesives containing sodium borate. Sodium borate concentration of 12–20% of the adhesive's total weight is equivalent to 2.6–5.3% boron. Because at least a portion of a dental adhesive is ingested, this amount of boron could cause chronic toxicity in denture wearers.

Denture Adhesive (Polyacrylamide polymer, modified cationic) A Class III device that is applied to the base of a denture before the denture is inserted into the patient's mouth. The device is used to improve denture retention and comfort.

Denture Adhesive (Polyvinylmethylether maleic acid calcium-sodium double salt) A Class I device that is applied to the base of a denture before the denture is inserted into the patient's mouth. The device is used to improve denture retention and comfort.

Denture Adhesive (Polyvinylmethylether maleic acid calcium-sodium double salt and carboxymethylcellulose sodium) A Class I device that is applied to the base of a denture before the denture is inserted into the patient's mouth. The device is used to improve denture retention and comfort.

Denture Relining, Repairing, or Rebasing Resin A Class II device composed of materials, such as methyl methacrylate, that are used to reline a denture surface that contacts tissue, to repair a fractured denture, or to form a new denture base. This device is not available over-the-counter.

Depth Gauge for Clinical Use A Class I measuring device intended for various medical purposes, such as to determine the proper length of screws for fastening the ends of a fractured bone.

Desoxycorticosterone Test System A Class I device intended to measure desoxycorticosterone (DOC) in plasma and urine. DOC measurements are used in the diagnosis and treatment of patients with hypermineralocorticoidism (excess retention of sodium and loss of potassium) and other disorders of the adrenal gland.

Device Any instrument, apparatus, implement, machine, contrivance, implant, in vitro reagent, or other similar or related article including any component part, or accessory.

Device (Antistammering device) A Class I device that electronically generates a noise when activated or when it senses the user's speech and that is intended to prevent the user from hearing the sounds of his or her own voice. The device is used to minimize a user's involuntary hesitative or repetitive speech.

Device, Biofeedback A Class II device that provides a signal corresponding to the status of the patient's physiological parameters (brain alpha waves, muscle activity, skin temperature, etc.) so that the patient can voluntarily control these parameters.

Device, Biopsy A Class II device used to remove samples of tissue for diagnostic purposes.

Device, Bleeding Time A Class II device usually employing two spring-loaded blades that produce two small incisions in the skin. The length of time required for the bleeding to stop is a measure of the effectiveness of the coagulation system, particularly the platelets.

Device, Blood Access A Class II device intended to provide access to the blood for hemodialysis or equivalent uses.

Device History Record (Regulatory) A compilation of records containing the complete production history of a finished device.

Device Master Record (Regulatory) A compilation of records containing the design, formulation, specifications, complete manufacturing procedures, quality assurance requirements, and labelling of a finished device.

Device (Calibrator) for Red Cell and White Cell Counting A Class II device that approximates whole blood or red or white blood cells, and that is used to set instruments intended to count red cells, white cells, or both. It is a suspension of particles or fixed cells whose size, shape, concentration and other characteristics have been carefully determined.

Devices for Sealing Microsections A Class I device that is an automated instrument used to seal stained cells and microsections for histological and cytological examination.

Diagnostic Computer (Programmable) A Class II device that can be programmed to compute various physiologic or blood-flow parameters on the output from one or more electrodes, transducers, or measuring devices. This device includes any associated commercially supplied programs.

Diagnostic Computer (Single-Function, preprogrammed) A Class II device composed of a hard-wired computer that calculates a specific physiological or blood-flow parameter based on information obtained from one or more electrodes, transducers, or measuring devices.

Diagnostic Condensing Lens A Class I device used in binocular indirect ophthalmoscopy (a procedure that produces an inverted or reversed direct magnified image of the eye) intended to focus reflected light from the fundus of the eye.

Diagnostic Electromyograph A Class II device used to monitor and display the bioelectric signals produced by muscles, to stimulate peripheral nerves, and to monitor and display the electrical activity produced by nerves for the diagnosis and prognosis of neuromuscular disease.

Diagnostic Electromyograph Needle Electrode A Class II monopolar or bipolar needle that is inserted into muscle or nerve tissue to sense bioelectric signals. The device is used in conjunction with diagnostic electromyography (recording the intrinsic electrical properties of skeletal muscle).

Diagnostic Hruby Fundus Lens A Class I device that is a 55 diopter lens intended for use in the examination of the vitreous body and the fundus of the eye under slitlamp illumination and magnification.

Diagnostic Intravascular Catheter A Class II device used to record intracardiac pressures, to sample blood, and to introduce substances into the heart and vessels. Included in this generic group are right-heart catheters, left-heart catheters, and angiographic catheters, among others.

Diagnostic Muscle Stimulator A Class II device use mainly with an electromyograph machine to initiate muscle activity and is used to diagnose and/or treat motor nerve or sensory neuromuscular disorders and neuromuscular function.

Diagnostic Pulmonary-Function Interpretation Calculator A Class II diagnostic anesthesiology device that interprets pulmonary study data used to determine the clinical significance of pulmonary-function tests.

Diagnostic Ultrasonic Transducer A Class II device made of a piezoelectric material that converts electrical signals into acoustic signals and acoustic signals into electrical signals and is intended for use in diagnostic ultrasonic medical devices. Accessories of this generic type of device may include transmission media for acoustically coupling the transducer to the body surface, such as acoustic gel, paste, or a flexible fluid container.

Diagnostic X-ray Beam-Limiting Device A Class II device, such as a collimator, a cone, or an aperture, intended to restrict the dimensions of a diagnostic X-ray field by limiting the size of the primary X-ray beam.

Diagnostic X-ray High Voltage Generator   A Class II device that is intended to supply and control the electrical energy applied to a diagnostic X-ray tube for medical purposes. This generic type of device may include a converter that changes alternating current to direct current, filament transformers for the X-ray tube, high-voltage switches, electrical protective devices, or other appropriate elements.

Diagnostic X-ray Tube Housing Assembly   A Class II device that is an X-ray generating tube encased in a radiation-shielded housing that is intended for diagnostic purposes. This generic type of device may include high voltage and filament transformers or other appropriate components.

Diagnostic X-ray Tube Mount   A Class II device intended to support and to position the diagnostic X-ray tube housing assembly for a medical radiographic procedure.

Differential Culture Medium   A Class I device that consists primarily of liquid and/or solid biological materials used to cultivate and indentify different types of microorganisms. The identification of these microorganisms is accomplished by the addition of a specific biochemical component(s) to the medium. Microorganisms are identified by a visible change (e.g., a color change) in a specific biochemical component(s) that indicates that specific metabolic reactions have occurred. Test results aid in the diagnosis of disease and also provide epidemiological information on diseases caused by these microorganisms.

Differential Pressure Transducer   A Class II two-chambered device used during pulmonary function testing. It generates an electrical signal for subsequent display or processing that is proportional to the difference in gas pressures in the two chambers.

Digitoxin Test System   A Class II device intended to measure digitoxin, a cardiovascular drug, in serum and plasma. Measurements obtained by this device are used in the diagnosis and treatment of digitoxin overdose and in monitoring levels of digitoxin to ensure appropriate therapy.

Digoxin Test System   A Class II device intended to measure digoxin, a cardiovascular drug, in serum and plasma. Measurements obtained by this device are used in the diagnosis and treatment of digoxin overdose and in monitoring levels of digoxin to ensure appropriate therapy.

Dilator (Esophageal)   A Class II device that consists of a cylindrical instrument that may be hollow and weighed with mercury or a metal, olive-shaped weight that slides on a guide, such as a string or wire, and is used to dilate a stricture of the esophagus. This generic type of device includes esophageal or gastrointestinal bougies and the esophageal dilator.

Dilator (Rectal) A Class II device designed to dilate the anal sphincter and canal when the size of the anal opening may interfere with its function or the passage of the examining instrument.

Dilator (Urethral) A Class II device that consists of a specially shaped catheter or bougie and is used to dilate the ureter at the place where a stone has become lodged or to dilate a ureteral stricture.

Diphenylhydantoin Test System A Class II device intended to measure diphenylhydantoin, an antiepileptic drug, in human specimens. Measurements obtained by this device are used in the diagnosis and treatment of diphenylhydantoin overdose and in monitoring levels of diphenylhydantoin to ensure appropriate therapy.

2,3-Diphosphoglyceric Acid Test System A Class I device intended to measure 2,3-diphosphoglyceric acid (2,3-DPG) in erythrocytes (red blood cells). Measurements of 2,3-diphosphoglyceric acid are used in the diagnosis and treatment of blood disorders that affect the delivery of oxygen by erythrocytes to tissues and in monitoring the quality of stored blood.

Discrete Photometric Chemistry Analyzer for Clinical Use A Class I device intended to duplicate manual analytical procedures by performing automatically various steps such as pipetting, preparing filtrates, heating, and measuring color intensity. This device is intended for use in conjunction with certain materials to measure a variety of analytes. Different models of the device incorporate various instrumentation such as microanalysis apparatus, double beam, single, or dual channel photometers, and bichromatic 2-wavelength photometers. Some models of the device may include reagent-containing components that may also serve as reaction units.

Dislodger (Ureteral stone) A Class II device that consists of a bougie or a catheter with an expandable wire basket near the tip, a special flexible tip, or other special construction. It is inserted through a cystoscope and used to entrap or remove stones from the lower ureter. This generic type of device includes the metal basket and the flexible ureteral stone dislodger.

Disposable Fluoride Tray A Class I device made of styrofoam that is used for the topical application of fluoride to the teeth. To employ the tray, the patient bites down on the tray that has been filled with a fluoride solution.

Distometer A Class I device intended to measure the distance between the cornea and a corrective lens during refraction to help measure the change of the visual image when a lens is in place.

Drape Adhesive A Class I device intended to be placed on the skin to attach a surgical drape.

Dressing (Absorbable hemostatic agent and dressing) A Class III device intended to produce hemostasis by accelerating the clotting process of blood. It is absorbable.

Dye or Chemical Solution Stains Class I devices which are either solutions of one or more synthetic and/or natural dyes or solutions of one or more nondye chemicals used to stain cells and tissue for diagnostic histopathology and hematology.

Dye Powder Stains Class I devices that are either synthetic or natural dyes used in the staining of cells and tissues for diagnostic histopathology and hematology.

E

Ear, Nose, and Throat Bur A Class I device consisting of an interchangeable drill bit that is intended for use in an ear, nose, and throat electric or pneumatic surgical drill for incising or removing bone in the ear, nose, or throat area. The bur consists of a carbide cutting tip on a metal shank or a coating of diamond on a metal shank. The device is used in mastoid surgery, frontal sinus surgery, and surgery of the facial nerves.

Ear, Nose, and Throat Drug Administration Device A Class I device that is one of a group of ear, nose, and throat devices intended specifically to administer medicinal substances to treat ear, nose, and throat disorders. These instruments include the powder blower, dropper, ear wick, manual nebulizer pump, and nasal inhaler.

Ear, Nose, and Throat Electric or Pneumatic Surgical Drill A Class II rotating, drilling device, including the handpiece, that is intended to drive various accessories, such as an ear, nose, and throat bur, for the controlled incision or removal of bone in the ear, nose, and throat area.

Ear, Nose, and Throat Examination and Treatment Unit An AC-powered Class I device intended to support a patient during an otologic examination while providing specialized features for examination and treatment. The unit consists of a patient chair and table, drawers for equipment, suction and blowing apparatus, and receptacles for connection of specialized lights and examining instruments.

Ear, Nose, and Throat Fiberoptic Light Source and Carrier An AC-powered Class II device that generates and transmits light through glass of plastic fibers and that is intended to provide illumination at the tip of an ear, nose, or throat endoscope. Endoscope devices which utilize fiberoptic light sources and carriers include the bronchoscope, esophagoscope, laryngoscope, mediastinoscope, laryngeal-bronchial telescope, and nasopharyngoscope.

Ear, Nose, and Throat Manual Surgical Instrument One of a variety of Class I devices intended for use in surgical procedures to examine or treat the bronchus, esophagus, trachea, larynx, pharynx, nasal and paranasal sinus, or ear. This generic type of device includes the esophageal dilator; tracheal bistour (a long, narrow surgical knife); tracheal dilator; tracheal hook, laryngeal injection set—laryngeal knife; laryngeal saw; laryngeal trocar; laryngectomy tube; adenoid curette; adenotome; metal tongue depressor; mouth gag; oral screw; salpingeal curette, tonsillotome; tonsile guillotine; tonsil screw, tonsil snare; tonsil suction tub; tonsil suturing hook; anatomic perforator; ethmoid curette; frontal sinus-rasp; nasal curette; nasal rasp; nasal rongeur; nasal saw; nasal scissors; nasal snare; sinus irrigator; sinus trephine; ear curette; ear excavator; ear rasp; ear scissor; ear snare; ear spoon; ear suction tub; malleous ripper; mastoid gauge; microsurgical ear chisel; myringotomy tube inserter; ossici holding clamp; sacculotomy tack inserter; vein press; wire ear loop; microrule; mirror; mobilizer; ear, nose, and throat punch; ear, nose, and throat knife; and ear, nose, and throat trocar.

Ear, Nose, and Throat Microsurgical Carbon Dioxide Laser A Class II device intended for the surgical excision of tissue from the ear, nose, and throat area. The device is used, for example, in microsurgical procedures to excise lesions and tumors of the vocal cords and adjacent areas.

Ear, Nose, and Throat Synthetic Polymer Material A Class II device material that is intended to be implanted for use as a space-occupying substance in the reconstructive surgery of the head and neck. The device is used, for example, in augmentation rhinoplasty and in tissue defect closures in the esophagus. The device is shaped and formed by the surgeon to conform to the patient's needs. This generic type of device is made of material such as polyamide mesh or foil and porous polyethylene.

Ear Oximeter A Class II extravascular device used to transmit light at known wavelengths through blood in the ear. The amount of reflected or scattered light as indicated by this device is used to measure the blood oxygen saturation.

Ear Prosthesis A Class II silicon rubber solid device intended to be implanted in order to reconstruct the external ear.

Earphone Cushion for Audiometric Testing A Class I device that is used to cover an audiometer earphone during audiometric testing to provide an acoustic coupling (sound connection path) between the audiometer earphone and the patient's ear.

***Echinococcus* spp. Serological Reagents**   Class I devices that consist of *Echinococcus* spp. antigens and antisera used in serological tests to identify *Echinococcus* spp. antibodies in a patient's serum. The identification aids in the diagnosis of echinococcosis, which is caused by parasitic tapeworms belonging to the genus *Echinococcus*, and provides epidemiological information on this type of disease. Echinococcosis is characterized by the development of cysts formed by the larva of the infecting organism in the liver, lung, kidneys and other organs.

Echocardiograph   A Class II device that uses ultrasonic energy to create images of cardiovascular structures. It includes phased arrays and two-dimensional scanners.

Echovirus Serological Reagents   Class I devices that consist of antigens and antisera used in serological tests to identify echovirus antibodies in a patient's serum. Additionally, some of these reagents consist of echovirus antisera conjugated with a fluorescent dye used to identify echoviruses from clinical specimens and/or from tissue culture isolates derived from clinical specimens. The identification aids in the diagnosis of echovirus infections and provides epidemiological information on diseases caused by these viruses. Echoviruses cause illnesses such as meningitis (inflammation of the brain and spinal cord membranes), febrile illnesses (accompanied by fever) with or without rash, and the common cold.

Elbow Joint Humeral (Hemi-elbow) Metallic Uncemented Prosthesis   A Class III device intended to be implanted and is made of alloys, such as cobalt-chromium-molybdenum. It is used to replace the distal end of the humerus formed by the trochlea humeri and the capitulum humeri. This generic type of device is limited to prostheses intended for use without bone cement.

Elbow Joint Metal/Metal or Metal/Polymer Constrained Cemented Prosthesis   A Class III device intended to be implanted to replace an elbow joint. It is made exclusively of alloys, such as cobalt-chromium-molybdenum, or made from these alloys with an ultra-high molecular weight polyethylene bushing. The device prevents dislocation in more than one anatomic plane and consists of two components that are linked together. This generic type of device is limited to those prostheses intended for use with bone cement.

Elbow Joint Metal/Polymer Semiconstrained Cemented Prosthesis   A Class II device intended to be implanted to replace an elbow joint. The device limits translation and rotation in one or more planes via the geometry of its articulating surfaces. It has no linkage across-the-joint. This generic type of device includes prostheses that consist of a humeral resurfacing component made of alloys, such as cobalt-chromium-molybdenum, and a radial resurfacing component made of ultra-high molecular weight polyethylene. This generic type of device is limited to those prostheses intended for use with bone cement.

Elbow Joint Radial (Hemi-elbow) Polymer Prosthesis   A Class II device intended to be implanted to replace the proximal end of the radius. It is made of medical-grade silicone elastomer.

Electric Positioning Chair   A Class II device with a motorized positioning control that can be adjusted to various positions. The device is used to provide stability for patients with athetosis (involuntary spasms) and to alter postural positions for therapeutic purposes.

Electric Powered Percussor   A Class II device used to transmit vibration through a patient's chest wall to aid in freeing mucus deposits in the lung in order to improve bronchial drainage.

Electrical Peripheral Nerve Stimulator   A Class II device (peripheral nerve stimulator or neuromuscular blockade monitor) used to apply an electrical current to a patient to test the level of pharmacological effect of anesthetic drugs and gases.

Electrically Powered Oxygen Tent   A Class II device that encloses the patient's head and, via an electrically powered unit, administers inspiratory oxygen and provides control of the temperature and humidity. This generic type of device also includes the pediatric aerosol tent.

Electroanesthesia Apparatus   A Class II device used for the induction and maintenance of anesthesia during surgical procedures by means of an alternating or pulsed electric current that is passed through electrodes fixed in the patient's head.

Electrocardiograph   A Class II device used to process the electrical signal transmitted through two or more ECG electrodes and to produce a visual display of the electrical signal produced by the heart.

Electrocardiograph Conducting Media   A Class II device consisting of the conducting jelly or paste that is applied to the surface of the body to transmit the electrical signal at the body surface to the electrocardiograph (ECG) electrode.

Electrocardiograph Electrode   A Class II device connector which is applied to the surface of the body to transmit the electrical signal on the body surface to a processor that produces an electrocardiogram or vectorcardiogram.

Electrocardiograph Lead Switching Adaptor   A Class II device composed of a passive switching device to which ECG limb and chest leads may be attached. This device is used to connect various com-

Electroconvulsive Therapy Device

binations of limb and chest leads to the output terminals in order to create standard lead combinations such as leads I, II, and III.

Electroconvulsive Therapy Device A Class II device used for treating severe psychiatric disturbances, e.g., severe depression, by inducing a major motor seizure through a brief intensive electrical current delivered to the head.

Electrode, Cutaneous A Class II device used to record physiological signals, or to apply electrical stimulation.

Electrode, Depth A Class II device used for temporary stimulation, or recording electrical signals at subsurface levels of the brain.

Electrode Cable A Class I device composted of strands of insulated electrical conductors laid together around a central core and used to connect an electrode from a patient to a diagnostic machine.

Electrode Gel for Pulp Tester A Class I device that is applied to the surface of a tooth before use of a pulp tester to aid conduction of electrical current.

Electroencephalographic Monitor A Class II device used to detect, measure, and graphically record the rhythmically varying electrical skin potentials produced by the fetal brain. This is accomplished by placing electrodes transcervically on the fetal scalp during labor.

Electroglottograph An AC-powered Class II device that employs a pair of electrodes that are placed in contact with the skin on both sides of the larynx and held in place by a collar. It is intended to measure the electrical impedance of the larynx to aid in assessing the degree of closure of the vocal cords, confirm laryngeal diagnosis, aid behavioral treatment of voice disorders, and aid research concerning the laryngeal mechanism.

Electrohydraulic Lithotriptor A Class III AC-powered device used to fragment urinary bladder stones. It consists of a high-voltage source connected by a cable to a bipolar electrode that is introduced into the urinary bladder through a cystoscope. With the bladder full of water, the electrode is held against the stone and repeated electrical discharges between the two poles of the electrode cause electrohydraulic shock waves which disintegrate the stone.

Electromyograph A Class II device used to monitor and display the bioelectric signals produced by muscles for the diagnosis and prognosis of neuromuscular disease.

Electronic Metal Locator An AC-powered Class II device with probes intended to locate metallic foreign bodies in the eye or eye socket.

Electronic Noise Generator for Audiometric Testing A Class II device that consists of a swept frequency generator, an amplifier, and an earphone. It is intended to introduce a masking noise into the nontest ear during an audiometric evaluation. The device minimizes the nontest ear's sensing of test tones and signals being generated for the ear being tested.

Electronic Vision Aid An AC-powered or battery-powered Class I device that consists of an electronic sensor/transducer intended for use by a patient who has impaired vision or blindness to translate visual images of objects into tactile or auditory signals.

Electrophoresis Apparatus for Clinical Use A Class I device intended to separate molecules or particles, including plasma proteins, lipoproteins, enzymes, and hemoglobins on the basis of their net charge in specified buffered media. This device is used in conjunction with certain materials to measure a variety of analytes as an aid in the diagnosis and treatment of certain disorders.

Electrophoretic Hemoglobin Analysis System A Class II device that electrophoretically separates and identifies normal and abnormal hemoglobin types as an aid in the diagnosis of anemia or erythrocytosis (increased total red cell mass) due to a hemoglobin abnormality.

Electrostatic X-ray Imaging System A Class II device intended for medical purposes that uses an electrostatic field across a semiconductive plate, a gas-filled chamber, or other similar device to convert a pattern of X-radiation into an electrostatic image and, subsequently, into a visible image. This generic type of device may include signal analysis and display equipment, patient and equipment supports, component parts, and accessories.

Electrosurgical Cutting and Coagulation Device and Accessories A Class II device intended to remove tissue and control bleeding by use of high-frequency electrical current.

Embolectomy Catheter A Class II device that is a balloon-tipped catheter used to remove thromboemboli that have migrated from blood vessels from one site in the vascular tree to another.

Emergency Airway Needle A Class II device used to puncture the cricothyroid membrane to provide an emergency airway during upper airway obstruction.

Emergency Ventilator A Class II device used to provide emergency respiratory support via a face mask, or a tube inserted in a patient's airway.

Emission Computed Tomography System A Class II device intended to detect the location and distribution of gamma ray- and positron-emitting radionuclides in the body and produce cross-sectional images through computer reconstruction of the data. This generic type of device may include signal analysis and display equipment, patient and equipment supports, radionuclide anatomical markers, component parts, and accessories.

Endocervical Aspirator   A Class II device designed to remove tissue from the endocervix (mucous membrane lining the canal of the uterine cervix) by suction with a syringe, bulb and pipette, or catheter. This device is used to evaluate the endocervical tissue to detect malignant and premalignant lesions.

Endodontic Dry Heat Sterilizer   A Class III device used to sterilize endodontic and other dental instruments by the application of dry heat. The heat is supplied through glass beads which have been heated by electricity.

Endodontic Paper Point   A Class I device made of paper that is used during endodontic therapy to dry, or apply medication to, the root canal of a tooth.

Endodontic Silver Point   A Class I device made of silver that is used during endodontic therapy to fill permanently the root canal of a tooth.

Endodontic Stabilizing Splint   A Class II device made of a material, such as titanium, that is used to stabilize a tooth by inserting the device through the root canal and into the upper or lower jaw bone.

Endolymphatic Shunt   A Class II device that consists of a tube or sheet intended to be implanted to relieve the symptoms of vertigo. The device permits the unrestricted flow of excess endolymph from the distended end of the endolymphatic system into the mastoid cavity where resorption occurs. This device is made of polytetrafluoroethylene or silicone elastomer.

Endolymphatic Shunt Tube with Valve   A Class III device that consists of a pressure-limiting valve associated with a tube intended to be implanted in the inner ear to relieve the symptoms of vertigo. The device directs excess endolymph from the distended end of the endolymphatic system into the mastoid cavity where resorption occurs. The function of the pressure-limiting inner ear valve is to impede the flow of endolymph so that a physiologically normal endolymphatic pressure is maintained. The device is made of silicone elastomer and polyamide and contains gold radiopaque markers within the silicone elastomer sheath.

Endometrial Aspirator   A Class II device designed to remove tissue from the endocervix by suction with a syringe, bulb, pipette, or catheter. It is used to evaluate endocervical tissue in order to detect malignant and premalignant tissue.

Endometrial Brush   A Class III device designed to remove samples of the endometrium (the mucosal lining of the uterus) by brushing its surface. This device is used to study endometrial cytology (cells).

Endometrial Suction Curette and Accessories A Class II device designed to remove material from the mucosal lining of the uterus by scraping and vacuum suction. This device is used for biopsy or menstrual extraction. This generic type of device may include catheters, syringes, and tissue filters or traps. The Panel previously considered this generic type of device under the name "endometrial suction biopsy curette."

Endometrial Washer A Class III device used to remove materials from the endometrium (the mucosal lining of the uterus) by washing with water or saline solution under negative pressure. This device is used to study endometrial cytology (cells).

Endomyocardial Biopsy Device A Class II device used to remove samples of tissue from the inner wall of the heart.

Endoscope A device used to provide access, illumination, observation, and manipulation of body cavities, hollow organs, and canals. Examples are: endoscopes, anoscopes, pneumoperitoneoscopes, choledoscopes, colonoscopes, cystoscopes, cystourethroscopes, esophagogastroduodenoscopes, esophagoscopes, pancreatoscopes, proctoscopes, resectoscopes, nephroscopes, sigmoidoscopes, transcervical scopes, urethroscopes, and accessories.

Endoscopic Electrosurgical Unit and Accessories A Class II device used to perform electrosurgical procedures through an endoscope. This generic type of device includes the electrosurgical generator, patient plate, electric biopsy forceps, electrode, flexible snare, electrosurgical alarm system, electrosurgical power supply unit, electrical clamp, self-opening rigid snare, flexible suction coagulator electrode, patient return wristlet, contact jelly, adaptor to the cord for transurethral surgical instruments, the electric cord for transurethral surgical instruments, and the transurethral desiccator.

Endoscopy The naked eye inspection of body cavities by means of tubular illuminated optical instruments. The most frequently used types of endoscopes are listed below.

Type	Range of Use	Example
Bronchoscope	Trachea	Tumors
Cardioscope	Heart cavities	Valvular and septal defects
Cystoscope	Urinary bladder	Tumors, stones, inflammation
Esophagoscope	Esophagus	Bleeding, tumors
Gastroscope	Stomach	Gastritis, ulcers, tumors
Laparoscope	Abdomen	Tumors
Laryngoscope	Larynx	Inflammation, tumors
Ophthalmoscope	Eye fundus	Retinal detachment, vessels

Type	Range of Use	Example
Otoscope	Tympanic membrane	Infections, perforations
Proctoscope	Rectum	Hemorrhoids, tumors
Sigmoidoscope	Rectum, colon	Diverticulosis, tumors
Thorascope	Pleural cavity air	Tumors

Endosseous Implant A Class III device of a material, such as titanium, that is surgically placed in the bone of the upper or lower jaw arches to provide support for prosthetic devices, such as artificial teeth, and to restore the patient's chewing function.

Enema Kit A Class I device intended to instill water or other fluids into the colon through a nozzle inserted into the rectum in order to promote evacuation of the contents of the lower colon. The device consists of a container for fluid connected to the nozzle either directly or via tubing.

Enflurane Gas Analyzer A Class II diagnostic anesthesiology device used to measure the concentration of enflurane anesthetic in a gas mixture.

Enriched Culture Medium A Class I device that consists primarily of liquid and/or solid biological materials used to cultivate and identify fastidious microorganisms (having complex nutritional requirements). The device consists of a relatively simple basal medium enriched by the addition of such nutritional components as blood, blood serum, vitamins, and extracts of plant or animal tissues. The device is used in the diagnosis of disease caused by pathogenic microorganisms and also provides epidemiological information on these diseases.

***Entamoeba histolytica* Serological Reagents** Class I devices that consist of antigens and antisera used in serological tests to identify *Entamoeba histolytica* antibodies in a patient's serum. Additionally, some of these reagents consist of antisera conjugated with a fluorescent dye (immunofluorescent reagents) used to identify *Entamoeba histolytica* directly from clinical specimens. The identification aids in the diagnosis of amebiasis caused by the microscopic protozoan parasite *Entamoeba histolytica* and provides epidemiological information on diseases caused by this parasite. The parasite may invade the skin, liver, intestines, lungs, and diaphragm, causing disease conditions such as indolent ulcers, amebic hepatitis, amebic dysentery, and pulmonary lesions.

Enuresis Alarm A Class II device used in the treatment of bedwetting. Through an electrical trigger mechanism, the device sounds an alarm when a small quantity of urine is detected on a sensing pad. This generic type of device includes the conditioned response enuresis alarm.

Environmental Chamber for Storage of Platelet Concentrate A Class

II device used to hold platelet-risk plasma within a preselected temperature range.

Enzyme Analyzer for Clinical Use   A Class I device intended to measure enzymes in plasma or serum by nonkinetic or kinetic measurement of enzyme-catalyzed reactions. This device is used in conjunction with certain materials to measure a variety of enzymes as an aid in the diagnosis and treatment of certain enzyme-related disorders.

Enzyme Preparations   Class I device products that are used in the histopathology laboratory for the following purposes: (1) to disaggregate tissues and cells already in established cultures for preparation into subsequent cultures (e.g., trypsin); (2) to disaggregate fluid specimens for cytological examination (e.g., papain for gastric lavage or trypsin for sputum liquefaction); (3) to aid in the selective staining of tissue specimens (e.g., diastase for glycogen determination).

Epilator (Needle-type epilator)   A Class II device intended to destroy the dermal papilla of a hair by applying electric current at the tip of a fine needle that has been inserted close to the hair shaft, under the skin, and into the dermal papilla. The electric current may be high-frequency AC current, high-frequency AC combined with DC current, or DC current only.

Epilator (Tweezer-type epilator)   An electrical Class III device intended for hair removal. The device provides a high-frequency electric current at the tip of a tweezer used for removing hair.

Epistaxis Balloon   A Class I device consisting of an inflatable balloon intended to control internal nasal bleeding by exerting pressure against the sphenopalatine artery.

Epstein-Barr Virus Serological Reagents   Class I devices that consist of antigens and antisera used in serological tests to identify Epstein-Barr virus antibodies in a patient's serum. The identification aids in the diagnosis of Epstein-Barr virus infections and provides epidemiological information on diseases caused by this virus. Epstein-Barr virus is thought to cause the infectious mononucleosis and has been associated with Burkitt's lymphoma (a tumor of the jaw in African children and young adults) and postnasal carcinoma.

Equine Encephalomyelitis Virus Serological Reagents   Class I devices that consist of antigens and antisera used in serological tests to identify equine encephalitis virus antibodies in a patient's serum. The identification aids in the diagnosis of diseases caused by equine encephalomyelitis viruses and provides epidemiological information on these viruses. Equine encephalomyelitis viruses are transmitted to humans by the bite of insects, such as mosquitos and ticks, and may cause encephalitis (inflammation of the brain), rash, acute arthritis, or hepatitis.

***Erysipelothrix rhusiopathiae* Serological Reagents** Class I devices that consist of antigens and antisera used in serological tests to identify *Erysipelothrix rhusiopathiae* from cultured isolates derived from clinical specimens. The identification aids in the diagnosis of disease caused by this bacterium belonging to the genus *Erysipelothrix*. This organism is responsible for a variety of skin inflammations following skin abrasions from contact with fish, shellfish, or poultry.

Erythrocyte Glucose-6-phosphate Dehydrogenase Assay A Class II device used to measure the activity of the enzyme glucose-6-phosphate dehydrogenase or of glucose-6-phosphate dehydrogenase isoenzymes. The results of this assay are used in the diagnosis and treatment of nonspherocytic congenital hemolytic anemia or drug-induced hemolytic anemia associated with a glucose-6-phosphate dehydrogenase deficiency. This generic device includes assays based on fluorescence, electrophoresis, methemoglobin reduction, catalase inhibition, and ultraviolet kinetics.

Erythrocyte Sedimentation Rate Test A Class I device that measures the length of time required for the red cells in a blood sample to fall a specified distance. An increased rate indicates tissue damage or inflammation.

Erythropoietin Assay A Class III device that measures the concentration of erythropoietin (an enzyme that regulates the production of red blood cells) in serum or urine. This assay provides diagnostic information for the evaluation of erythrocytosis (increased total red cell mass) and anemia.

***Escherichia coli* Serological Reagents** Class I devices that consist of antigens and antisera used in serological tests to identify *Escherichia coli* from cultured isolates derived from clinical specimens. Additionally, some of these reagents consist of *Escherichia coli* antisera conjugated with a fluorescent dye used to identify *Escherichia coli* directly from clinical specimens and/or cultured isolates derived from clinical specimens. The identification aids in the diagnosis and treatment of disease caused by this bacterium belonging to the genus *Escherichia* and provides epidemiological information on diseases caused by this microorganism. Although *Escherichia coli* constitutes the greater part of the microorganisms found in the intestinal tract in humans and is usually nonpathogenic, those strains that are pathogenic may cause urinary tract infections and/or epidemic diarrheal disease, especially in children.

Esophageal Dilator A Class II device that consists of a cylindrical instrument that may be hollow and weighed by mercury or a metal olive-shaped weight that slides on a guide, such as a string or wire, and is used to dilate a stricture of the esophagus. This generic type of device includes esophageal or gastrointestinal bougies and the esophageal dilator.

Esophageal Obturator A Class II device inserted through the patient's mouth to facilitate ventilation of the patient during emergency resuscitation by occluding the esophagus, thereby permitting positive pressure ventilation through the trachea. The device consists of a closed-end semirigid esophageal tube that is attached to a face mask.

Esophageal Prosthesis A plastic tube or tube-like Class III device that may have mesh reinforcement that is intended to be implanted in, or affixed externally to, the chest and throat to restore the esophagus or provide pharyngoesophageal continuity.

Esophageal Stethoscope with Electrical Conductors A Class II diagnostic anesthesiology device that is inserted into the esophagus to listen to heart and breath sounds and to monitor electrophysiological signals. The device may also incorporate a thermistor for temperature measurement.

Esophagoscope (Flexible or rigid) and Accessories A tubular endoscopic Class II device with any of a group of accessory devices that attached to the esophagoscope. It is intended to examine or treat esophageal malfunction symptoms, esophageal or mediastinal disease, or to remove foreign bodies from the esophagus. When inserted, the device extends from the area of the hypopharynx to the stomach. It is typically used with a fiberoptic light source and carrier to provide illumination. The device is made of materials such as stainless steel or flexible plastic. This generic type of device includes the flexible foreign body claw, flexible biopsy forceps, rigid biopsy curette, flexible biopsy brush, rigid biopsy forceps, and flexible biopsy curette, but excludes the fiberoptic light source and carrier.

Estradiol Test System A Class I device intended to measure estradiol, an estrogenic steroid, in plasma. Estradiol measurements are used in the diagnosis and treatment of various hormonal sexual disorders and in assessing placental function in a complicated pregnancy.

Estriol Test System A Class I device intended to measure estriol, an estrogenic steroid, in plasma, serum, and urine of pregnant females. Estriol measurements are used in the diagnosis and treatment of fetoplacental distress in certain cases of high-risk pregnancy.

Estrogens (Total, in pregnancy) Test System A Class I device intended to measure total estrogens in plasma, serum, and urine during pregnancy. The device primarily measures estrone plus estradiol. Measurements of total estrogens are used to aid in the diagnosis and treatment of fetoplacental distress in certain cases of high-risk pregnancy.

Estrogens (Total, nonpregnancy) Test System A Class I device intended to measure the level of estrogens (total estrone, estradiol, and estriol) in plasma, serum, and urine of males and nonpregnant females. Measurement of estrogens (total, nonpregnancy) is used in the diagnosis and treatment of numerous disorders, including infertility, amenorrhea (absence of menses) differentiation of primary and secondary ovarian malfunction, estrogen secreting testicular and ovarian tumors, and precocious puberty in females.

Estrone Test System A Class I device intended to measure estrone, an estrogenic steroid, in plasma. Estrone measurements are used in the diagnosis and treatment of numerous disorders, including infertility, amenorrhea, differentiation of primary and secondary ovarian malfunction, estrogen secreting testicular and ovarian tumors, and precocious puberty in females.

Ether Hook A Class II device that fits inside the patient's mouth and is used to deliver vaporized ether.

Ethosuximide Test System A Class II device intended to measure ethosuximide, an antiepileptic drug, in human specimens. Measurements obtained by this device are used in the diagnosis and treatment of ethosuximide overdose and in monitoring levels of ethosuximide to ensure appropriate therapy.

Etiocholanolone Test System A Class I device intended to measure etiocholanolone in serum and urine. Etiocholanolone is a metabolic product of the hormone testosterone and is excreted in the urine. Etiocholanolone measurements are used in the diagnosis and treatment of disorders of the testes and ovaries.

Euglobulin Lysis Time Test A Class II device that measures the length of time required for the lysis (dissolution) of a clot formed from fibrinogen in the euglobulin fraction (that fraction of the plasma responsible for the formation of plasmin, a clot-lysing enzyme). This test evaluates natural fibrinolysis (destruction of a blood clot after bleeding has been arrested). The test will detect accelerated fibrinolysis.

Euthyscope A Class I device that is a modified AC-powered or battery-powered ophthalmoscope (a perforated mirror device intended to inspect the interior of the eye) that projects a bright light encompassing an arc of about 30° onto the fundus of the eye. The center of the light bundle is blocked by a black disk covering the fovea (the central depression of the macular retinae where only cones are present and blood vessels are lacking). The device is intended for use in the treatment of amblyopia (dimness of vision without apparent disease of the eye). Note: Class I for the battery-powered device. Class II for the AC-powered device.

Evacuator (Gastroenterology-urology) A Class II device used to remove debris and fluids during gastroenterological and urological procedures by drainage, aspiration, or irrigation. This generic type of device includes the fluid evacuator system, manually operated bladder evacuator, and the AC-powered vacuum pump.

Exercise Component A Class I device that is used in conjunction with exercise equipment or with other forms of exercise. Examples of an exercise component include a weight, a dumbbell, a strap, and a hand mitt.

Exophthalmometer A Class I device, such as a ruler gauge, or caliper, intended to measure the degree of exophthalmos (abnormal protrusion of the eyeball).

Expandable Cervical Dilator A Class III instrument with two handles and two opposing blades used manually to dilate (stretch open) the cervix.

External Aesthetic Restoration Prosthesis A Class I device intended to be used to construct an external artificial body structure, such as an ear, breast, or nose. Usually the device is made of silicone rubber and it may be fastened to the body with an external prosthesis adhesive. The device is not intended to be implanted.

External Assembled Limb Prosthesis A Class II, preassembled external artificial limb for the lower extremity. Examples of external assembled lower limb prostheses are the following: knee/shank/ankle/foot assembly and thigh/knee/shank/ankle/foot assembly.

External Cardiac Compressor A Class III device that is electrically, pneumatically, or manually powered and is used to compress the chest periodically in the region of the heart to provide blood flow during cardiac arrest.

External Counterpulsating Device A Class III device used to assist the heart by applying positive or negative pressure to one or more of the body's limbs in synchrony with the heart cycle.

External Facial Fracture Fixation Appliance A Class I metal apparatus intended to be used during surgical reconstruction and repair to immobilize maxillofacial bone fragments in their proper facial relationship.

External Limb Orthotic Component A Class I device used in conjunction with an orthosis (brace) to increase the function of the orthosis for a patient's particular needs. Examples of external limb orthotic component include the following: a brace-setting twister and an external brace stirrup.

External Limb Overload Warning Device A powered Class II device used to warn a patient of an overload or an underload in the amount of pressure placed on a leg.

External Limb Prosthetic Components A Class I device that, when put together with other appropriate components, constitutes a total prosthesis. Examples of external limb prosthetic components include the following: ankle, foot, hip, knee, and socket components; mechanical or powered hand; hook; wrist unit; elbow joint; and shoulder joint components and cable, and prosthesis suction valves.

External Nasal Splint   A rigid or partially rigid Class I device intended for use externally for immobilization of parts of the nose.

External Pacemaker Pulse Generator   A Class III device that has a power supply and electronic circuits that produce electrical pulses to stimulate the heart. This device, which is used outside the body, is used as a temporary substitute for the heart's intrinsic pacing system until a permanent pacemaker can be implanted, or to control irregular heartbeats in patients following cardiac surgery or a myocardial infarction. The device may have adjustments for impulse strength, duration, R-wave sensitivity, and other pacing variables.

External Prosthesis Adhesive   A Class I device composed of a silicone-type adhesive intended to be used to fasten to the body an external aesthetic restoration prosthesis, such as an artificial nose.

External Transcutaneous Cardiac Pacemaker   A Class III device used to supply a periodic electrical impulse intended to pace the heart. The device is usually applied to the surface of the chest through electrodes, such as defibrillator paddles.

External Uterine Contraction Monitor and Accessories (1133)   A Class II device used to monitor the progress of labor. It measures the strength, duration, and frequency of uterine contractions with a transducer strapped to the maternal abdomen. This generic type of device may include external pressure transducer, support straps, and other patient and equipment supports.

External Vein Stripper   A Class II device used to remove a section of a diseased vein.

Extraocular Orbital Implant   A nonabsorbable Class II device intended to be implaned during scleral surgery for buckling or building up the floor of the eye, usually in conjunction with retinal reattachment. Injectable substances are excluded.

Extraoral Orthodontic Headgear   A Class I device that is used, in conjunction with an orthodontic applicance, to exert pressure on the teeth from outside the mouth. The headgear has a strap that wraps around the patient's neck or head and an inner bow portion that is fastened to the orthodontic appliance in the patient's mouth.

Extraoral Source X-ray System   A Class II device that produces X-rays and is used for dental radiographic examination and diagnosis of diseases of the teeth, jaw, and oral structures. The X-ray source is located outside the mouth. This generic type of device may include patient and equipment supports and component parts.

Extravascular Blood Flow Probe   A Class II device ultrasonic or electromagnetic probe used in conjunction with a blood flowmeter to measure blood flow in a chamber or vessel.

Extravascular Blood Pressure Transducer   A Class II device used to measure blood pressure by changes in mechanical or electrical properties of the device. The proximal end of the transducer is connected to a pressure monitor that produces analog or digital electrical signals paralleling changes in blood pressure.

Eye Movement Monitor   An AC-powered Class II device with an electrode intended to measure and record ocular movements.

Eye Pad   A Class I device that consists of a pad made of various materials, such as gauze and cotton, intended for use as a bandage over the eye for protection or absorption of secretions.

Eye Sphere Implant   A Class II device intended to be implanted in the eyeball to occupy space following the removal of the contents of the eyeball with the sclera left intact.

Eye Valve Implant   A one-way, pressure-sensitive, valve-like Class III device intended to be implanted to normalize intraocular pressure. The device may be used in the treatment of glaucoma.

F

Facebow   A Class I device used in denture fabrication to determine the spatial relationship between the upper and lower jaws. This determination is used to place denture casts accurately into an articulator (a device that holds a set of plaster dental casts and reproduces jaw movements) and thereby aids the correct placement of artificial teeth into the denture base.

Factor XIII, A, S, Immunological Test System   A Class I device that consists of the reagents used to measure, by immunochemical techniques, the factor XIII (a blood-clotting factor) in platelets (A) or serum (S). Measurements of factor XIII, A, S, aid in the diagnosis of certain bleeding disorders resulting from a deficiency of this factor.

Fallopian Tube Prosthesis   A Class II device designed to maintain the patency (openness) of the fallopian tube and is used after reconstructive surgery.

Fatty Acids Test System   A Class I device intended to measure fatty acids in plasma and serum. Measurements of fatty acids are used in the diagnosis and treatment of various disorders of lipid metabolism.

FDA   Abbreviation for Food and Drug Administration, the agency formed in 1931 under the Department of Health, Education, and Welfare (HEW), that is concerned with the safety and efficacy of products marketed for medical use. The FDA also promulgates interstate commerce regulations. Under this broad mandate, the regulatory powers of the FDA have been steadily expanding by congressional acts, such as the Food, Drug, and Cosmetics (FD&C) Act of 1938, the Radiological Products Act of 1971, the Toxicological Research Act of 1972, and the Medical Device Amendment Act of 1976. The most respected regulatory agency in the federal government, it is estimated that in 1988 the FDA's annual operating cost reached $1.85 per consumer.

FDA, Device Statutes   Regulations and their governing statutes that pertain to medical device biomaterials are listed below:

(1) Recognized in the official *National Formulary,* the *United States Pharmacopeia,* or any supplement to these publications

(2) Intended for use in the diagnosis of disease or other condition, or in the cure, mitigation, treatment, or prevention of disease, in man or other animals

(3) Intended to affect the structure or any function of the body of man or other animals

(4) Does not achieve any of its principal intended purposes through chemical action within or on the body of man or other animals and that is not dependent on being metabolized for the achievement of any of its principal intended purposes

(5) Pre-1976 devices that were subsequently classified into Class III, and devices that are substantially equivalent to these devices

(6) Pre-1976 devices that were regulated as new drugs

(7) Post-1976 devices that are not substantially equivalent to devices commercially available before the Medical Device Amendments were enacted

Ferritin Immunological Test System   A Class II device that consists of the reagents used to measure, by immunochemical techniques, the ferritin (an iron storing protein) in serum and body fluids. Measurements of ferritin aid in the diagnosis of diseases affecting iron metabolism, such as hemochromatosis (iron overload) and iron deficiency anemia.

Fetal Blood Sampler   A Class II device used to obtain fetal blood transcervically through an endoscope by puncturing the fetal skin with a short blade and drawing blood into a heparinized tube. The fetal blood pH is determined and used in the diagnosis of fetal distress and fetal hypoxia.

Fetal Cardiac Monitor A Class II device designed to separate fetal heart signals from maternal heart signals by analyzing electrocardiographic signals (electrical potentials generated during contraction and relaxation of heart muscle) obtained from the maternal abdomen with external electrodes or from another monitor. The device is used to ascertain fetal heart activity during pregnancy and labor. This generic type of device may include an alarm that signals when the heart rate crosses a preset threshold.

Fetal Electroencephalographic Monitor A Class III device used to detect, measure and record in graphic form (by means of one or more electrodes placed transcervically on the fetal scalp during labor) the rhythmically varying electrical skin potentials produced by the fetal brain.

Fetal Hemoglobin Assay A Class II device that is used to determine the presence and distribution of fetal hemoglobin (hemoglobin F) in red cells or to measure the amount of fetal hemoglobin present. The assay may be used to detect fetal red cells in the maternal circulation or to detect elevated levels of fetal hemoglobin in hemoglobin abnormalities such as thalassemia (a hereditary hemolytic anemia characterized by decreased synthesis of one or more types of hemoglobin polypeptide chain). The hemoglobin determination may be made by means of such methodologies as electrophoresis, alkali denaturation, column chromatography, and radial immunodiffusion.

Fetal Phonocardiographic Monitor and Accessories A Class III device designed to detect, measure, and record fetal heart sounds electronically, in graphic form, and noninvasively, to ascertain fetal condition during labor. This generic type of device includes the following accessories: signal analysis and display equipment, patient and equipment supports, and other component parts.

Fetal Scalp Circular (Spiral) Electrodes and Applicator A Class II obstetrical device used to obtain a fetal electrocardiogram during labor and delivery. It establishes electrical contact between fetal skin and an external monitoring device by a shallow subcutaneous puncture of fetal scalp tissue with a curved needle or needles. This device includes nonreusable spiral electrodes and reusable circular electrodes.

Fetal Scalp Clip Electrode and Applicator A Class III device designed to establish electrical contact between fetal skin and an external monitoring device by means of pinching skin tissue with a non-reusable clip. This device is used to obtain a fetal electrocardiogram. This generic type of device may include a clip electrode applicator.

Fetal Stethoscope   A Class I device used for listening to fetal heart sounds. It is designed to transmit the fetal heart sounds not only through sound channels by air conduction but also through the user's head by tissue conduction into the user's ears. It does not use ultrasonic energy. This device is designed to eliminate noise interference commonly caused by handling conventional stethoscopes.

Fetal Ultrasonic Monitor and Accessories   A Class II device designed to transmit and receive ultrasonic energy into and from the pregnant woman, usually by means of continuous wave (doppler) echoscopy. The device is used to represent some physiological condition or characteristic as a measure value over a period of time (e.g., perinatal monitoring during labor), or in an immediately perceptible form (e.g., use of the ultrasonic stethoscope). This generic type of device includes the folowing accessories: signal analysis and display equipment, electronic interfaces for other equipment, patient and equipment supports, and component parts. This generic type of device does not include devices (imagers) used to monitor some relatively unchanging physiological condition, but does include devices which may be set to alarm automatically at a predetermined threshold value.

Fetal Vacuum Extractor   A Class II obstetric device used to facilitate delivery. It applies traction to the fetal head (in the birth canal) by means of a suction cup attached to the scalp and is powered by an external vacuum source. This generic type of device may include the vacuum source and vacuum control.

Fiber (Medical absorbent)   A Class I device made from cotton or synthetic fiber in the shape of a ball or pad used for applying medication to, or absorbing small amounts of fluids from, the patient's body surface.

Fiberoptic Dental Light   A Class I AC-powered device, usually attached to a dental handpiece, that consists of glass or plastic fibers that have optical properties. The device is used to illuminate oral structures.

Fiberoptic Light Ureteral Catheter   A Class II device that consists of a fiberoptic bundle that emits light throughout its length and is shaped so that it can be inserted into the ureter to enable the path of the ureter to be seen during lower abdominal or pelvic surgery.

Fiberoptic Oximeter Catheter   A Class II device used to estimate the oxygen saturation of the blood. It consists of two fiberoptic bundles that conduct light at a desired wavelength through blood and detect the reflected and scattered light at the distal end of the catheter.

Fibrin Monomer Procoagulation Test   A Class II device used to detect fibrin monomer in the diagnosis of disseminated intravascular coagulation (nonlocalized clotting within a blood vessel) or in the differential diagnosis between disseminated intravascular coagulation and primary fibrinolysis (dissolution of the fibrin in a blood clot).

Fibrin Split Products Assay   A Class II device used to detect and quantitate fibrin split products (protein fragments produced by the enzymatic action of plasmin on fibrin) as an aid in detecting the presence and degree of intravascular coagulation and fibrinolysis (the dissolution of the fibrin in a blood clot) and in monitoring therapy for disseminated intravascular coagulation (nonlocalized clotting in the blood vessels).

Fibrinogen Determination System   A Class II device that consists of the instruments, reagents, standards, and controls used to determine the fibrinogen levels in disseminated intravascular coagulation (nonlocalized clotting within the blood vessels) and primary fibrinolysis (the dissolution of fibrin in a blood clot).

Fibrinopeptide A Immunological Test System   A Class II device that consists of the reagents used to measure, by immunochemical techniques, the fibrinopeptide A (a blood-clotting factor) in plasma and body fluids. Measurement of fibrinopeptide A may aid in the diagnosis and treatment of certain blood-clotting disorders.

Filter (Cardiovascular intravascular)   A Class II implanted device placed in the inferior vena cava for the purpose of preventing pulmonary thromboemboli from flowing into the right side of the heart and the pulmonary circulation.

Finger Joint Metal/Metal Constrained Cemented Prosthesis   A Class III device intended to be implanted to replace a metacarpophalangeal (finger) joint. This device prevents dislocation in more than one anatomic plane and has components which are linked together. This generic type of device includes prostheses that are made of alloys such as cobalt-chromium-molybdenum, and is limited to those prostheses intended for use with bone cement.

Finger Joint Metal/Metal Constrained Uncemented Prosthesis   A Class III device intended to be implanted to replace a metacarpophalangeal or proximal interphalangeal (finger) joint. The device prevents dislocation in more than one anatomic plane and consists of two components that are linked together. This generic type of device includes prostheses made of alloys, such as cobalt-chromium-molybdenum, or prostheses made from alloys and ultra-high molecular weight polyethylene. This generic type of device is limited to prostheses intended for use without bone cement.

Finger Joint Metal/Polymer Constrained Cemented Prosthesis   A Class III device intended to be implanted to replace a metacarpophalangeal or proximal interphalangeal (finger) joint. The device prevents dislocation in more than one anatomic plane, and consists of two components that are linked together. This generic type of device includes prostheses that are made of alloys such as cobalt-chromium-molybdenum and ultra-high molecular weight polyethylene, and is limited to those prostheses intended for use with bone cement.

Finger Joint Polymer Constrained Prosthesis A Class II device intended to be implanted to replace a metacarpophalangeal or proximal interphalangeal (finger) joint. This generic type of device includes prostheses that consist of a single flexible across-the-joint component made from either a silicone elastomer or a combination of polypropylene and polyester material. The flexible across-the-joint component may be covered with a silicone rubber sleeve.

Finished Device A device, or an accessory to a device, that is suitable for use whether or not it is packaged or labelled for commercial distribution.

Fixation Device An AC-powered Class I device intended for use as a fixation target for the patient during ophthalmological examination. The patient directs his or her gaze so that the visual image of the object falls on the fovea centralis (the center of the macular retina of the eye).

Flame Emission Photometer for Clinical Use A Class I device intended to measure the concentration of sodium, potassium, lithium, and other metal ions in body fluids. Abnormal variations in the concentration of these substances in the body are indicative of certain disorders (e.g., electrolyte imbalance and heavy metal intoxication) and are, therefore, useful in diagnosis and treatment of those disorders.

***Flavobacterium* spp. Serological Reagents** Class I devices that consist of antigens and antisera used in serological tests to identify *Flavobacterium* spp. from cultured isolates derived from clinical specimens. The identification aids in the diagnosis of disease caused by bacteria belonging to the genus *Flavobacterium* and provides epidemiological information on diseases caused by these microorganisms. Most members of this genus are found in soil and water and, under certain conditions, may become pathogenic to humans. *Flavobacterium* meningosepticum is highly virulent for the newborn, in whom it may cause epidemics of septicemia (blood poisoning) and meningitis (inflammation of the membranes of the brain) and is usually attributable to contaminated hospital equipment.

Flexible Diagnostic Fresnel Lens A Class I device that is a very thin lens that has on its surface a concentric series of increasingly refractive zones. The device is intended to be applied to the back of the spectacle lenses of patients with aphakia (absence of the lens of the eye).

Flotation Cushion   A Class I device made of plastic that is filled with water, air, gel, or mud, and is used on a seat to lessen the likelihood of skin ulcers.

Flowmeter (Bourdon gauge)   A Class II device used in conjunction with respiratory equipment to sense gas pressure. The device is calibrated to indicate gas flow rate with the outflow open to the atmosphere.

Flowmeter (Compensated Thorpe tube)   A Class II device used to indicate and control gas flow rate accurately. The device includes a vertically mounted tube and is calibrated when the outlet of the flowmeter is attached to a reference pressure.

Flowmeter (Gas calibration)   A Class II device used to calibrate flowmeters and accurately measure gas flow.

Flowmeter (Uncompensated Thorpe tube)   A Class II device used to indicate and control gas flow rate accurately. The device includes a vertically mounted tube and is calibrated when the outlet of the flowmeter is open to the atmosphere.

Fluorescent Scanner   A Class II device intended to measure the induced fluorescent radiation in the body by exposing the body to certain X-rays or low-energy gamma rays. This generic type of device may include signal analysis and display equipment, patient and equipment supports, component parts, and accessories.

Fluorometer for Clinical Use   A Class I device intended to measure, by fluorescence, certain analytes. Fluorescence is the property of certain substances of radiating, when illuminated, a light of a different wavelength. This device is used in conjunction with certain materials to measure a variety of analytes.

Folic Acid Test System   A Class II device intended to measure the vitamin folic acid in plasma and serum. Folic acid measurements are used in the diagnosis and treatment of megaloblastic anemia, which is characterized by the presence of megaloblasts (an abnormal red blood cell series) in the bone marrow.

Follicle-Stimulating Hormone Test System   A Class I device intended to measure follicle-stimulating hormone (FSH) in plasma, serum, and urine. FSH measurements are used in the diagnosis and treatment of pituitary gland and gonadal disorders.

Food and Drug Act   Originally passed in 1906 to regulate the purity and safety of foods and drugs. In 1938, Congress passed the Federal Food, Drug, and Cosmetic Act, which required manufacturers of new drugs to prove safety for premarketing approval of new drugs. In 1962, the act was amended to provide regulatory authority to assure both safety and efficacy of all new drugs.

Force-Measuring Platform (1189) A Class II device that converts pressure applied upon a planar surface into analog mechanical or electrical signals. This device is used to determine ground reaction force, centers of percussion, centers of torque, and their variations in both magnitude and direction with time.

Forceps for Articulation Paper A Class I device used to hold articulation paper in the proper position between the upper and lower teeth when the teeth are in the bite position. The articulation paper locates uneven or high areas.

Forceps for a Rubber Dam Clamp A Class I plier-like device used to spread a rubber dam clamp (a device used to anchor a rubber dam in place) during insertion and removal of the clamp.

Forceps for Dental Dressing A Class I hand-held, tweezer-like device used to apply dressings to areas in the mouth during dental procedures.

Formiminoglutamic Acid (FIGLU) Test System A Class I device intended to measure formiminoglutamic acid in urine. FIGLU measurements obtained by this device are used in the diagnosis of anemias, such as pernicious anemia and congenital hemolytic anemia.

Fornixscope A Class I device intended to pull back and hold open the eyelid to aid examination of the conjunctiva.

***Francisella tularensis* Serological Reagents** Class II devices that consist of antigens and antisera used in serological tests to identify *Francisella tularensis* antibodies in a patient's serum and/or to identify *Francisella tularensis* in cultured isolates derived from clinical specimens. Additionally some of these reagents consist of antisera conjugated with a fluorescent dye (immunofluorescent reagents) used to identify *Francisella tularensis* directly from clinical specimens and/or cultured isolates derived from clinical specimens. The identification aids in the diagnosis of tularemia caused by *Francisella tularensis* and provides epidemiological information on this disease. Tularemia is a disease principally of rodents, but may be transmitted to humans through handling of infected animals, animal products, or by the bites of fleas and ticks. The disease takes on several forms depending upon the site of infection, such as skin lesions, lymph node enlargements, or pulmonary infection.

Free Secretory Component Immunological Test System A Class II device that consists of the reagents used to measure, by immunochemical techniques, free secretory component (normally a portion of the secretory IgA antibody molecule) in human body fluids. Measurement of free secretory component (protein molecules) aids in the diagnosis of persons with repetitive lung infections and other hypogammaglobulinemic conditions (low antibody levels).

Free Thyroxine Test System A Class II device intended to measure free (not protein bound) thyroxine (thyroid hormone) in serum or plasma. Levels of free thyroxine in plasma are thought to reflect the amount of thyroxine hormone available to the cells and may therefore determine the clinical metabolic status of thyroxine. Measurements obtained by this device are used in the diagnosis and treatment of thyroid diseases.

Free Tyrosine Test System A Class I device intended to measure free tyrosine (an amino acid) in serum and urine. Measurements obtained by this device are used in the diagnosis and treatment of diseases such as congenital tyrosinemia (a disease that can cause liver/kidney disorders) and as an adjunct to the measurement of phenylalanine in detecting congenital phenylketonuria (a disease that can cause brain damage).

Fusion and Stereoscopic Target A Class I device intended for use as a viewing object with a stereoscope.

G

Galactose Test System A Class I device intended to measure galactose in blood and urine. Galactose measurements are used in the diagnosis and treatment of the hereditary disease galactosemia (a disorder of galactose metabolism) in infants.

Galactose-1-phosphate Uridyl Transferase Test System A Class II device intended to measure the activity of the enzyme galactose-phosphate uridyl transferase in erythrocytes (red blood cells). Measurements of galactose-1-phosphate uridyl transferase are used in the diagnosis and treatment of the hereditary disease galactosemia (disorder of galactose metabolism) in infants.

Gas Collection Vessel A Class II diagnostic anesthesiology device used to collect a patient's exhaled gases for subsequent analysis. The device does not include a sampling pump.

Gas Cylinder A Class II device used as a container for pressurized medical gas. This identification applies only to gas containers that are empty, i.e., to containers that are not filled with gas by the manufacturer or distributor. A cylinder is considered empty when the pressure level is one tenth (1/10) of the labelled filling pressure at 21°C (70°F).

Gas Cylinder Holder A Class II device used to hold a gas cylinder in place.

Gas Flow Transducer A Class II device used to convert gas flow rate into an electrical signal for subsequent display or processing.

79

Gas Generating Device A Class I device that produces predetermined amounts of selected gases to be used in a closed chamber in order to establish suitable atmospheric conditions for cultivation of microorganisms with special atmospheric requirements. The device aids in the diagnosis of disease.

Gas Liquid Chromatography System for Clinical Use A Class I device intended to separate one or more drugs or compounds from a mixture. Each of the constituents in a vaporized mixture of compounds is separated according to its vapor pressure. The device may include accessories, such as columns, gases, column supports, and liquid coating.

Gas Pressure Regulator A Class II device used to calibrate pressure measuring instruments by generating a known gas pressure.

Gas Pressure Transducer A Class II device used to convert gas pressure into an electrical signal for subsequent display or processing.

Gas Scavenging Apparatus A Class II device used to collect excess anesthetic, analgesic, and trace gases and vapors from a breathing system, ventilator, or extracorporeal pump-oxygenator, and conduct these gases out of the personnel area by means of an exhaust system.

Gas Volume Calibrator A Class II diagnostic anesthesiology device used to calibrate the output of gas volume measurement instrumentation by delivering a known gas volume.

Gas-Powered Jet Injector A Class II device consisting of a syringe used to administer a local anesthetic. The syringe is powered by a cartridge containing pressurized carbon dioxide which provides the pressure to force the anesthetic out of the syringe.

Gastric Acidity Test System A Class I device intended to measure the acidity of gastric fluid. Measurements of gastric acidity are used in the diagnosis and treatment of patients with peptic ulcer Zollinger-Ellison syndrome (peptic ulcer due to a gastrin-secreting tumor of the pancreas), and related gastric disorders.

Gastrin Test System A Class I device intended to measure the hormone gastrin in plasma and serum. Measurements of gastrin are used in the diagnosis and treatment of patients with ulcers, pernicious anemia, and the Zollinger-Ellison syndrome (peptic ulcer due to a gastrin-secreting tumor of the pancreas).

Gastroenterology-Urology Biopsy Instrument A Class II device used to remove, by cutting or aspiration, a specimen of tissue for microscopic examination. This generic type of device includes the biopsy punch, gastrointestinal mechanical biopsy instrument, suction biopsy instrument, gastrourology biopsy needle and needle set, and nonelectric biopsy forceps. This recommendation does not apply to biopsy instruments that have specialized uses in other medical speciality areas and that were the subject of recommendation by other device classification panels.

Gastroenterology-Urology Evacuator A Class II device used to remove debris and fluids during gastroenterological and urological procedures by drainage, aspiration, or irrigation. This generic type of device includes the fluid evacuator system, manually operated bladder evacuator, and the AC-powered vacuum pump.

Gastroenterology-Urology Fiberoptic Retractor A Class I device that consists of a mechanical retractor with a fiberoptic light system that is used to illuminate deep surgical sites.

Gastroenterology-Urology Surgical Instrument and Accessories (Manual) A Class I device designed to be used for gastroentero-logical and surgical procedures. The device may be nonpowered, hand-held, or hand-manipulated. Manual instruments include the biopsy forceps cover, biopsy tray without biopsy instruments, line clamp, nonpowered rectal probe, nonelectrical clamp, needle holder, gastrourology hook, gastrourology probe and director, non-self-restraining retractor, laparotomy rings, nonelectrical snare, rec-tal specula, bladder neck spreader, self-restraining retractor, and scoop.

Gastrointestinal Mobility Monitoring System A Class II device used to measure peristaltic activity or pressure in the stomach or esopha-gus by means of a probe with transducers that is introduced through the mouth into the intestinal tract. The device may include signal conditioning, amplifying, and recording equipment. This generic type of device includes the esophageal motility monitor and tube, the gastrointestinal motility (electrical) system, and certain ac-cessories, such as a pressure transducer, amplifier, and external recorder.

Gastroscopy An examination with a lighted tube that enables in-spection of the stomach for abnormalities or disease conditions.

Gauge (Gas pressure) A Class II device used to measure the gas pressure in a gas delivery system. The gas pressure gauge may be of the Bourdon-type.

General Purpose Laboratory Equipment Labelled or Promoted for a Specific Medical Use A Class I device that is intended to prepare or examine specimens from the human body and that is labelled or promoted for a specific medical use.

General Purpose Reagent A Class I device composed of a chemical reagent that has general laboratory application. It is used to collect, prepare and examine specimens from the human body for diagnos-tic histopathology and hematology, and is not labelled or promoted for medical use or for a specific diagnostic application. General purpose reagents include cytological preservatives, decalcifying reagents, fixatives and adhesives, tissue processing reagents isotonic solutions, and pH buffers.

Genital Vibrator An electrically operated Class II device used to vibrate the female genitals as a form of massage in the treatment of sexual dysfunction and as an adjunct to Kegel's exercise (tightening of the muscles of the pelvic floor to increase muscle tone).

Gentamicin Test System A Class II device intended to measure gentamicin, an antibiotic drug, in human specimens. Measurements obtained by this device are used in the diagnosis and treatment of gentamicin overdose and in monitoring levels of gentamicin to ensure appropriate therapy.

Gingival Fluid Measurer A Class I device used to measure the amount of fluid in the gingival sulcus in order to determine if there is gingivitis disease.

Globulin Test System A Class I device intended to measure globulins (proteins) in plasma and serum. Measurements of globulin are used in the diagnosis and treatment of patients with numerous illnesses including severe liver and renal disease, multiple myeloma, and other disorders of blood globulins.

Glucagon Test System A Class I device intended to measure the pancreatic hormone glucagon in plasma and serum. Glucagon measurements are used in the diagnosis and treatment of patients with various disorders of carbohydrate metabolism, including diabetes mellitus, hypoglycemia, and hyperglycemia.

Glucose Test System A Class II device intended to measure glucose quantitatively in blood and other body fluids. Glucose measurements are used in the diagnosis and treatment of carbohydrate metabolism disorders including diabetes mellitus, neonatal hypoglycemia, and idiopathic hypoglycemia, and of pancreatic islet cell carcinoma.

γ-Glutamyl Transpeptidase and Isoenzymes Test System A Class I device intended to measure the activity of the enzyme gamma-glutamyl transpeptidase (GGTP) in plasma and serum. Gamma-glutamyl transpeptidase and isoenzymes measurements are used in the diagnosis and treatment of liver diseases, such as alcoholic cirrhosis and primary and secondary liver tumors.

Glutathione Reductase Assay A Class II device used to determine the activity of the enzyme glutathione reductase in serum, plasma, or erythrocytes by such techniques as fluorescence and photometry. The results of this test are used in the diagnosis of liver disease, glutathione reductase deficiency, or riboflavin deficiency.

Gluthathione Test System A Class I device intended to measure glutathione (the tripeptide of glycine, cysteine, and glutamic acid) in erythrocytes (red blood cells). Glutathione measurements are used in the diagnosis and treatment of certain drug-induced hemolytic (erythrocyte destroying) anemias due to an inherited enzyme deficiency.

β-2-Glycoprotein I Immunological Test System A Class I device that consists of the reagents used to measure, by immunochemical techniques, β-2-glycoprotein I (a serum protein) in serum and other body fluids. Measurement of β-2-glycoprotein I aids in the diagnosis of an inherited deficiency of this serum protein.

β-2-Glycoprotein III Immunological Test System A Class I device that consists of the reagents used to measure, by immunochemical techniques, the β-2-glycoprotein III (a serum protein) in serum and other body fluids. Measurement of β-2-glycoprotein III aids in the diagnosis of an inherited deficiency of this serum protein and a variety of other conditions.

α-2-Glycoproteins Immunological Test System A Class I device that consists of the reagents used to measure, by immunochemical techniques, the α-2-glycoproteins (a group of plasma proteins found in the α-2-group when subjected to electrophoresis) in serum and other body fluids. Measurement of α-2-glycoproteins aids in deficiencies of these plasma proteins.

GMPs (Good Manufacturing Practices) The primary basis on which the FDA evaluates a manufacturer's ability to produce a safe and effective device consistently. The Medical Device Amendments of 1976 expressly incorporated into the FDA act language authorizing the FDA to establish GMPs for the device industry. The FDA has promulgated regulations covering nearly all aspects of manufacturing—device components, production processes, production controls, packaging, storage, labelling, installation, and warehouse distribution procedures. These GMPs are intended to ensure that devices are safe and effective, and that they comply with statutory requirements. Two key documents for GMP compliance are the Center for Devices and Radiological Health (CDRH) May 1987 *Guidelines on Preproduction Quality Assurance and Process Validation*. These documents provide guidance on medical device product manufacturing. The purpose of GMPs is to provide a framework of manufacturing controls. The agency believes that manufacturers who adhere to these controls increase the probability that their device will conform to their established specifications. This means that if the medical device has been properly designed, following the GMPs will ensure that there is consistent manufacturing of that product with the appropriate quality control checks prior to its distribution and use.

Gold and Stainless Steel Cusp A Class I prefabricated device made of gold and stainless steel that provides a permanent cusp and is

83

used to achieve occlusal harmony between the teeth and a removable denture.

Gold-Based Alloy for Clinical Use   A Class II device that is a mixture of metals, the major component of which is gold. It may also contain smaller quantities of silver, copper, platinum, or palladium. It is used to fabricate custom-made dental appliances, such as crowns and bridges.

Goniometer   An AC-powered Class I device intended to evaluate joint function by measuring and recording ranges of motion, acceleration, or forces exerted by a joint.

Gonioscopic Prism   A Class I device that is a prism intended to be placed on the eye to study the anterior chamber. The device may have angled mirrors to facilitate visualization of anatomical features.

Group Hearing Aid or Group Auditory Trainer   A Class II hearing aid device that is intended for use in communicating simultaneously with one or more listeners having hearing impairment. The device is used with an associated transmitter microphone. It may be either monaural or binaural, and it provides coupling to the ear through either earphones or earmolds. The generic type of device includes three types of applications: hardwire systems, inductance loop systems, and wireless systems.

Guard for an Abrasive Disk   A Class I metal device that clips onto the dental handpiece. The guard shields soft tissue from injury by an abrasive disk when the disk is being used during construction of a restoration.

Gustometer   A battery-powered Class I device that consists of two electrodes that are intended to be placed on both sides of the tongue at different taste centers and that provides a galvanic stimulus resulting in taste sensation. It is used for assessing the sense of taste.

Gynecologic Electrocautery and Accessories   A device designed to destroy tissue with high temperatures by tissue contact with an electrically heated probe. It is used to excise cervical lesions, perform biopsies, or treat chronic cervicitis under direct visual observation. This generic type of device includes the following accessories: an electrical generator, a probe, and electrical cables.

Gynecologic Laparoscope and Accessories   A Class II device used to permit direct viewing of the organs within the peritoneum by a telescopic system introduced through the abdominal wall. It is used to perform diagnostic and surgical procedures on the female genital organs. This generic type of device may include trocar and cannula, instruments used through an operating channel, scope preheater, light source and cables, and component parts.

Gynecologic Surgical Laser   A Class II continuous wave, carbon dioxide laser device designed to destroy tissue thermally or to remove tissue by radiant light energy. This device is used only in conjunction with a colposcope as part of a gynecological surgical system. A colposcope is a magnifying lens system used to examine the vagina and cervix.

H

Haidlinger Brush An AC-powered Class I device that provides two conical, brush-like images with apexes touching that are viewed by the patient through a Nicol prism and intended to evaluate visual function. It may include a component for measuring macular integrity.

Halothane Gas Analyzer A Class II diagnostic anesthesiology device used to measure the concentration of Halothane anesthetic in a gas mixture. The device may use analytical techniques such as mass spectrometry or absorption of infrared and ultraviolet radiation.

Haploscope An AC-powered Class I device that consists of two movable viewing tubes, each containing a slide carrier, a low-intensity light source for the illumination of the slides, and a high-intensity light source for creating afterimages. The device is intended to measure strabismus (eye muscle imbalance), to assess binocular vision (use of both eyes to see), and to treat suppression and amblyopia (dimness of vision without any apparent disease of the eye).

Haptoglobulin Immunological Test System A Class II device that consists of the reagents used to measure, by immunochemical techniques, the haptoglobin (a protein that binds hemoglobin, the oxygen-carrying pigment in red blood cells) in serum. Measurement of haptoglobin may aid in the diagnosis of hemolytic diseases (diseases in which the red blood cells rupture and release hemoglobin) related to the formation of hemoglobin-haptoglobin complexes and certain kidney diseases.

Headband Mirror A Class I device intended to be strapped to the head of the user to reflect light for use in examination of the eye.

Hearing Aid A wearable, sound-amplifying Class I device that is intended to compensate for impaired hearing. This generic type of device includes the air-conduction hearing aid and the bone-conduction hearing aid, but excludes the group hearing aid or group auditory trainer.

Hearing Aid Calibrator and Analysis System An electronic reference Class II device intended to calibrate and assess the electroacoustic frequency and sound intensity characteristics emanating from a hearing aid, master hearing aid, group hearing aid, or group auditory trainer. The device consists of an acoustic complex of known cavity volume, a sound level meter, a microphone, oscillators, frequency counters, microphone amplifiers, a distoration analyzer, a chart recorder, and a hearing aid test box.

Heart Sound Transducer   A Class II device consisting of an external transducer that exhibits changes in mechanical or electrical properties in relation to cardiac sounds.

Heart Valve, Prosthetic, Holder   A Class II device used to hold a replacement heart valve while it is being sutured into place.

Heart Valve, Prosthetic, Sizer   A Class II device used to measure the size of the natural valve opening to determine the size of the appropriate replacement heart valve.

Heart Valve, Replacement   A Class III device intended to perform the function of any of the heart's natural valves. This generic device class includes valves constructed of prosthetic materials, biologic valves (e.g., porcine xenograft valves), or valves constructed of a combination of prosthetic and biologic materials.

Heat and Moisture Condenser (Artificial nose)   A Class II device positioned over a tracheotomy or tracheal tube to warm and humidify gases breathed by a patient.

Heat Sealing Device   A Class I device that uses heat to seal plastic bags containing blood or blood components.

Heat Source for Bleaching Teeth   A Class I AC-powered device used to apply heat to a tooth after the tooth is coated with a bleaching agent. The heat source may be either a light or an electric heater.

Heat Sterilizer   A Class II device that uses dry heat to sterilize medical products.

Helium Gas Analyzer   A Class II diagnostic anesthesiology device used to measure the concentration of helium in a gas mixture. The device may use analytical techniques such as thermal conductivity, gas chromatography, or mass spectrometry.

Hematocrit Measuring Device   A Class II device that is a system consisting of instruments, tubes, racks, a sealer, and a holder. The device is used to measure the packed red cell volume in blood to determine whether the patient's total red cell volume is normal or abnormal. Abnormal states include anemia (an abnormally low total red cell volume) and erythrocytosis (an abnormally high total red mass). The packed red cell volume is produced by centrifuging a given volume of blood.

Hematology Quality Control Mixture   A Class II device used to ascertain the accuracy and precision of manual, semiautomated, and automated determinations of cell parameters, such as white cell count (WBC), red cell count (RCC), platelet count (PLT), hemoglobin, hematocrit (HCT), mean corpuscular hemoglobin (MCH), and mean corpuscular hemoglobin concentration (MCHC).

Hematology Stains Class I devices composed of mixtures of synthetic or natural dyes, in solution, used in staining cells of peripheral blood and bone marrow on microscope slides for diagnostic hematology.

Hemoglobin A₂ Assay A Class II device used to determine the hemoglobin A_2 content of human blood. The measurement of hemoglobin A_2 is used in the diagnosis of the thalassemias (hereditary hemolytic anemias characterized by decreased synthesis of one or more types of hemoglobin polypeptide chain). Electrophoresis or column chromatography is used to make this measurement.

Hemoglobin Immunological Test System A Class II device that consists of the reagents used to measure, by immunochemical techniques, the different types of free hemoglobin (the oxygen-carrying pigment in red blood cells) in blood, urine, plasma, or other biological fluids. Measurement of free hemoglobin aids in the diagnosis of patients with various hematologic disorders, such as sickle cell anemia. Fanconi's anemia (a rare inherited disease), aplastic anemia (bone marrow does not produce enough blood cells), and leukemia (cancer of the blood-forming organs).

Hemolytic Immunological Test System A Class II device that consists of the reagents used to measure, by immunochemical techniques, immunoglobulins and C3 (the third component of complement) attached to the surface of a patient's red blood cells. Measurement of immunoglobulins and C3 on the surface of red blood cells aids in the diagnosis of hemolytic transfusion reactions (red cell destruction that results from a patient receiving blood from a noncompatible donor), hemolytic disease of the newborn (destruction of the red blood cells of an Rh + fetus of an Rh − mother), immune drug induced hemolytic anemia, such as a reaction to penicillin, as well as many autoimmune hemolytic anemias (destruction of red blood cells by the body's own antibodies) associated with chronic lymphocytic leukemia (cancer of the white blood cells), lymphoma (cancer of lymphoid tissues), systemic lupus erythematosus (a multisystem autoimmune disease), or paroxysmal nocturnal hemoglobinuria (hemoglobin in the urine).

Hemopexin Immunological Test System A Class II device that consists of the reagents used to measure, by immunochemical techniques, the hemopexin (a serum protein that binds heme, a component of hemoglobin) in serum. Measurement of hemopexin aids in the diagnosis of various hematologic disorders, such as hemolytic anemia (anemia due to shortened in vivo survival of mature red blood cells and inability of the bone marrow to compensate for their decreased life span) and sickle cell anemia.

***Hemophilus* spp. Serological Reagents** Class I devices that consist of antigens and antisera, including antisera conjugated with a fluorescent dye, that are used in serological tests to identify *Hemophilus* from cultured isolates derived from clinical specimens and/or directly from clinical specimens. The identification aids in the diagnosis of disease caused by bacteria belonging to the genus *Hemophilus* and provides epidemiological information on diseases caused by these microorganisms. Diseases most often caused by *Hemophilus* spp. include pneumonia, pharyngitis, sinusitis, vaginitis, chancroid veneral disease, and a contagious form of conjunctivitis (inflammation of eyelid membranes).

Hemorrhoidal Ligator A Class II device used to cut off the blood flow to hemorrhoidal tissue by means of a ligature or band placed around the hemorrhoid.

Heparin Assay A Class II device used to determine the level of the anticoagulant heparin in the patient's circulation. These assays are quantitative clotting time procedures utilizing the effect of heparin on activated coagulation factor X (Stuart factor) or procedures based on the neutralization of heparin by protamine sulfate (a protein that neutralizes heparin).

Herpes Simplex Virus Serological Reagents Class II devices that consist of antigens and antisera used in various serological tests to identify herpes simplex virus antibodies in a patient's serum. Additionally, some of these reagents consist of herpes simplex virus antisera conjugated with a fluorescent dye (immunofluorescent reagents) used to identify herpes simplex virus directly from clinical specimens and/or tissue culture isolates derived from clinical specimens. The identification aids in the diagnosis of diseases caused by herpes simplex viruses, and provides epidemiological information on these diseases. Herpes simplex viral infections range from common and mild lesions of the skin and mucous membranes to a severe form of encephalitis (inflammation of the brain).

High-Pressure Liquid Chromatography System for Clinical Use A Class I device intended to separate one or more drugs or compounds from a solution by processing the mixture of compounds (solutes) through a column packed with materials of uniform size (stationary phase) under the influence of a high-pressure liquid (mobile phase). Separation of the solutes occurs either by absorption, sieving, partition, or selective affinity.

Hip Joint (Hemi-hip) Acetabular Metal Cemented Prosthesis A Class III device intended to be implanted to replace a portion of the hip joint. This generic type of device includes prostheses that have an acetabular component made of alloys, such as cobalt-chromium-molybdenum. This generic type of device is limited to those prostheses intended for use with bone cement.

Hip Joint Femoral (Hemi-hip) Metal/Polymer Cemented or Uncemented Prosthesis A two-part Class II device intended to be implanted to replace the head and neck of the femur. This generic type of device includes prostheses that have a femoral component made of alloys, such as cobalt-chromium-molybdenum, and a snap-fit acetabular component made of an alloy, such as cobalt-chromium-molybdenum, and ultra-high molecular weight polyethylene. This generic type of device may be fixed to the bone with bone cement or implanted by impaction.

Hip Joint Femoral (Hemi-hip) Metallic Cemented or Uncemented Prosthesis A Class II device intended to be implanted to replace a portion of the hip joint. This generic type of device includes prostheses that have a femoral component made of alloys, such as cobalt-chromium-molybdenum. This generic type of device includes designs that are intended to be fixed to the bone with bone cement, as well as designs that have large, window-like holes in the stem of the device and that are intended for use without bone cement. However, in these latter designs, fixation of the device is not achieved by means of bone ingrowth.

Hip Joint Femoral (Hemi-hip) Metallic Resurfacing Prosthesis A Class II device intended to be implanted to replace a portion of the hip joint. This generic type of device includes prostheses that have a femoral resurfacing component made of alloys, such as cobalt-chromium-molybdenum.

Hip Joint Femoral (Hemi-hip) Trunnion-Bearing Metal/Polyacetal Cemented Prosthesis A two-part Class III device intended to be implanted to replace the head and neck of the femur. This generic type of device includes prostheses that consist of a metallic stem made of alloys, such as cobalt-chromium-molybdenum, with an integrated cylindrical trunnion bearing at the upper end of the stem that fits into a recess in the head of the device. The head of the device is made of polyacetal (polyoxymethylene), and it is covered by a metallic alloy, such as cobalt-chromium-molybdenum. The trunnion bearing allows the head of the device to rotate on its stem. The prosthesis is intended for use with bone cement.

Hip Joint Metal/Ceramic/Polymer Semiconstrained Cemented or Nonporous Uncemented Prosthesis A Class II device intended to be implanted to replace a hip joint. This device limits translation and rotation in one or more planes via the geometry of its articulating surfaces. It has no linkage across-the-joint. The two-part femoral component consists of a femoral stem made of alloys to be fixed in the intramedullary canal of the femur by impaction with or without use of bone cement. The proximal end of the femoral stem is tapered with a surface that ensures positive locking with the spherical ceramic (aluminum oxide, Al_2O_3) head of the femoral component. The acetabular component is made of ultra-high molecular weight polyethylene or ultra-high molecular weight polyethylene reinforced with nonporous metal alloys, and used with or without bone cement.

Hip Joint Metal/Composite Semiconstrained Cement Prosthesis A two-part Class II device intended to be implanted to replace a hip joint. The device limits translation and rotation in one or more planes via the geometry of its articulating surfaces. It has no linkage across-the-joint. This generic type of device includes prostheses that consist of a femoral component made of alloys, such as cobalt-chromium-molybdenum, and an acetabular component made of ultra-high molecular weight polyethylene with carbon fibers composite. Both components are intended for use with bone cement.

Hip Joint Metal/Polymer Constrained Cemented or Uncemented Prosthesis A Class III device intended to be implanted to replace a hip joint. The device prevents dislocation in more than one anatomic plane and has components that are linked together. This generic type of device includes prostheses that have a femoral component made of alloys, such as cobalt-chromium-molybdenum, and an acetabular component made of ultra-high molecular weight polyethylene. This generic type of device is intended for use with or without bone cement. This device is not intended for biological fixation.

Hip Joint Metal/Polymer Semiconstrained Cemented Prosthesis A Class II device intended to be implanted to replace a hip joint. The device limits translation and rotation in one or more planes via the geometry of its articulating surfaces. It has no linkage across-the-joint. This generic type of device includes prostheses that have a femoral component made of alloys, such as cobalt-chromium-molybdenum, and an acetabular resurfacing component made of ultra-high molecular weight polyethylene and is limited to those prostheses intended for use with bone cement.

Hip Joint Metal Constrained Cemented or Uncemented Prosthesis A Class III device intended to be implanted to replace a hip joint. The device prevents dislocation in more than one anatomic plane and has components that are linked together. This generic type of device includes prostheses that have components made of alloys, such as cobalt-chromium-molybdenum, and is intended for use with or without bone cement. This device is not intended for biological fixation.

Hip Joint Metal/Metal Semiconstrained, with an Uncemented Acetabular Component, Prosthesis A two-part Class III device intended to be implanted to replace a hip joint. The device limits translation and rotation in one or more planes via the geometry of its articulating surfaces. It has no linkage across-the-joint. This generic type of device includes prostheses that consist of a femoral and an acetabular component, both made of alloys, such as cobalt-chromium-molybdenum. The femoral component is intended to be fixed with bone cement. The acetabular component is intended for use without bone cement.

Hip Joint Metal/Metal Semiconstrained, with a Cemented Acetabular Component, Prosthesis A two-part Class III device intended to be implanted to replace a hip joint. The device limits translation and rotation in one or more planes via the geometry of its articulating surfaces. It has no linkage across-the-joint. This generic type of device includes prostheses that consist of a femoral and an acetabular component, both made of alloys, such as cobalt-chromium-molybdenum. This generic type of device is limited to those prostheses intended for use with bone cement.

Hip Joint Metal/Polymer Semiconstrained Resurfacing Cemented Prosthesis A two-part Class III device intended to be implanted to replace the articulating surfaces of the hip while preserving the femoral head and neck. The device limits translation and rotation in one or more planes via the geometry of its articulating surfaces. It has not linkage across-the-joint. This generic type of device includes prostheses that consist of a femoral cap component made of alloy, such as cobalt-chromium-molybdenum, that is placed over a surgically prepared femoral head, and an acetabular resurfacing polymer component. Both components are intended for use with bone cement.

Histidine Test System A Class I device intended to measure free histidine (an amino acid) in plasma and urine. Histidine measurements are used in the diagnosis and treatment of hereditary histidinemia characterized by excess histidine in the blood and urine often resulting in mental retardation and disordered speech development.

***Histoplasma capsulatum* Serological Reagents** Class II devices that consist of antigens and antisera used in serological tests to identify *Histoplasma capsulatum* antibodies in a patient's serum. Additionally, some of these reagents consist of *Histoplasma capsulatum* antisera conjugated with a fluorescent dye (immunofluorescent reagents) used to identify *Histoplasma capsulatum* from clinical specimens and/or culture isolates derived from clinical specimens. The identification aids in the diagnosis of histoplasmosis caused by this fungus belonging to the genus *Histoplasma* and provides epidemiological information on the diseases caused by this fungus.

Hot or Cold Disposable Pack A Class I device consisting of a sealed plastic bag incorporating chemicals that, upon activation, produces heat or cold. It is used when hot or cold therapy is indicated for body surfaces.

Human Allotypic Marker Immunological Test System   A Class I device that consists of the reagents used to identify by, immunochemical techniques, the inherited human protein allotypic markers (such as Gm2 and Km allotypes) in serum, saliva, and other biological fluids. The identification may be used while studying population genetics.

Human Chorionic Gonadotropin (HCG) Test Systems   (1) A Class II device intended for the early detection of pregnancy that measures HCG, a placental hormone, in plasma or urine. (2) A Class III device intended for any uses other than early detection of pregnancy (such as an aid in the diagnosis, prognosis, and management of treatment of persons with certain tumors or carcinomas) that measures HCG, a placental hormone, in plasma or urine.

Human Growth Hormone Test System   A Class I device intended to measure the levels of human growth hormone in plasma. Human growth hormone measurements are used in the diagnosis and treatment of disorders involving the anterior lobe of the pituitary gland.

Human Placental Lactogen Test System   A Class II device intended to measure the hormone human placental lactogen (HPL) [also known as human chorionic somatomammotrophin (HCS)], in maternal serum and maternal plasma. Measurements of human placental lactogen are used in the diagnosis and clinical management of high-risk pregnancies involving fetal distress associated with placental insufficiency. Measurements of HPL are also used in pregnancies complicated by hypertension, proteinuria, edema, postmaturity, placental insufficiency, or possible miscarriage.

Humidifier for Home Use   A Class II device used to add water vapor to inspired gases for respiratory therapy. The vapor produced by the device pervades the area surrounding the patient and is inspired during normal respiration.

Hydraulic Adjustable Hospital Bed   A Class I device consisting of a bed with a hydraulic mechanism operated by an attendant to adjust the height and surface contour of the bed. The device includes movable and latchable side rails.

Hydraulic, Pneumatic and Photoelectric Plethysmograph   A Class II device used to estimate blood flow in a region of the body using hydraulic, pneumatic, or photoelectric measurement techniques.

Hydrophilic Resin Coating for Dentures   A Class I device used to improve denture retention and comfort. The device consists of a water-retaining polymer cream that is applied to the base of a denture before the denture is inserted into the patient's mouth.

Hydroxybutyric Dehydrogenase Test System   A Class I device intended to measure the activity of the enzyme α-hydroxybutyric dehydrogenase (HBD) in plasma or serum. HBD measurements are used in the diagnosis and treatment of myocardial infarction, renal damage (such as rejection of transplants), certain hematological diseases (such as acute leukemias and megaloblastic anemias) and, to a lesser degree, liver disease.

17-Hydroxycorticosteroids (17-Ketogenic steroids) Test System A Class I device intended to measure corticosteroids possessing a dihydroxyacetone ($HOCH_2$–CO–CHO_2H) moiety on the steroid nucleus in urine. Corticosteroids with this chemical configuration include cortisol, cortisone 1,1-desoxycortisol, desoxycorticosterone, and their tetrahydro derivatives. This group of hormones is synthesized by the adrenal gland. Measurements of 17-hydroxycorticosteroids (17-ketogenic steroids) are used in the diagnosis and treatment of various diseases of the adrenal or pituitary glands and gonadal disorders.

5-Hydroxyindole Acetic Acid/Serotonin Test System A Class I device intended to measure 5-hydroxyindole acetic acid/serotonin in urine. Measurements of 5-hydroxyindole acetic acid/serotonin are used in the diagnosis and treatment of carcinoid tumors of endocrine tissue.

17-Hydroxyprogesterone Test System A Class I device intended to measure 17-hydroxyprogesterone (a steroid) in plasma and serum. Measurements of 17-hydroxyprogesterone are used in the diagnosis and treatment of various disorders of the adrenal glands or the ovaries.

Hydroxyproline Test System A Class I device intended to measure the amino acid hydroxyproline in urine. Hydroxyproline measurements are used in the diagnosis and treatment of various collagen (connective tissue) diseases, bone disease, such as Paget's disease, and endocrine disorders, such as hyperparathyroidism and hyperthyroidism.

Hygroscopic-Laminaria Cervical Dilator A Class II device designed to dilate (stretch open) the cervix by cervical insertion of a conical and expansible material made from the root of a seaweed (*Laminaria digitata*).

Hyperbaric Chamber A Class II device that can be pressurized to greater than atmospheric pressure. It is used to increase the environmental oxygen pressure to promote the movement of oxygen from the environment to the patient's tissue. This classification does not include those chambers used solely for topical applications.

Hypersensitivity Pneumonitis Immunological Test System A Class II device that consists of the reagents used to measure, by immunochemical techniques, the immunoglobulin antibodies which react specifically with organic dust derived from fungal or animal protein sources. When these antibodies react with such dusts in the lung, immune complexes precipitate and trigger an inflammatory reaction (hypersensitivity pneumonitis). Measurement of these immunoglobulin G antibodies aid in the diagnosis of hypersensitivity pneumonitis and other allergic respiratory disorders.

Hyperthermia Device   A Class II device composed of a soft, liquid-filled blanket and a heat exchanger that is used to warm all or part of the body.

Hysteroscope and Accessories   A Class II device used to permit direct viewing of the cervical canal and the uterine cavity by telescopic system introduced into the uterus through the cervix. It is used to perform diagnostic and surgical procedures other than sterilization. This generic type of device may include obturators and sheaths, instruments used through an operating channel, scope preheaters, light sources and cables, and component parts.

Hysteroscopic Insufflator   A Class II device designed to distend the uterus by filling the uterine cavity with a liquid or gas to facilitate viewing with a hysteroscope.

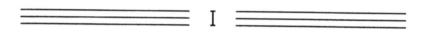

I

IDE (Investigational Device Exemptions)   The purpose is ". . . to encourage, to the extent consistent with the protection of the public health and safety and with ethical standards, the discovery and development of useful devices intended for human use and to that end to maintain optimum freedom for scientific investigators in their pursuit of that purpose." Without this section of the law, it would be impossible for device manufacturers to be in compliance with the law and at the same time provide for clinical testing to establish the safety and effectiveness of devices.

Image Intensification Vision Aid   A battery-powered Class I device to amplify ambient light that is intended for use by a patient who has limited dark adaptation or impaired vision.

Image-Intensified Fluoroscopic X-ray System   A Class II device intended to visualize anatomical structures by converting a pattern of X-radiation into a visible image through electronic amplification. This generic type of device may include signal analysis and display equipment, patient and equipment supports, component parts, and accessories.

Immersion Hydrobath   A Class II device consisting of an immersion hydrobath (e.g., whirlpool) with water agitators and may include a tub to be filled with water. The water temperature may be measured by a gauge. It is used in hydrotherapy to relieve pain and itching, and as an aid in the healing process of inflamed and traumatized tissue. It serves as a setting for removal of contaminated tissue.

Immunoelectrophoresis Equipment A Class I device for clinical use (with an electrical power supply) that separates protein molecules. Immunoelectrophoresis is a procedure in which a complex protein mixture is placed in an agar gel and the various proteins are separated on the basis of their relative mobilities under the influence of an electric current. The separated proteins are then permitted to diffuse through the agar toward a multispecific antiserum, allowing precipitation and visualization of the separate complexes.

Immunoephelometer Equipment (Includes immunologic test system) A Class I device for clinical use (with an electrical power supply) that measures light scattering from antigen-antibody complexes. The concentration of these complexes may be measured by means of reflected light. A beam of light passed through a solution is scattered by the particles in suspension. The amount of light is detected by a photo detector which converts light energy into electrical energy. The amount of electrical energy registers on a readout system, such as a digital voltmeter or a recording chart. This electrical readout is called the light-scattering value and is used to measure the concentration of antigen-antibody complexes.

Immunofluorometer Equipment (Includes U.V. immunologic test system) A Class I device for clinical use (with an electrical power supply) that measures the fluorescence of fluorochrome-labelled antigen-antibody complexes. The concentration of these complexes may be measured by means of reflected light. A beam of light is passed through a solution in which a fluorochrome has been selectively attached to serum protein antibody molecules in suspension. The amount of light emitted by the fluorochrome label is detected by a photodetector, which converts light energy into electrical energy. The amount of electrical energy registers on a readout system, such as a digital voltmeter or a recording chart. This electrical readout is called the fluorescence value and is used to measure the concentration of antigen-antibody complexes.

Immunoglobulin G (Fab Fragment specific) Immunological Test System A Class II device that consists of the reagents used to measure, by immunochemical techniques, the Fab antigen-binding fragment resulting from breakdown of immunoglobulin G antibodies in urine, serum, and other biological fluids. Measurement of Fab fragments of immunoglobulin G aids in the diagnosis of lymphoproliferative disorders, such as multiple myeloma (tumor of bone marrow cells), Waldenstrom's macroglobulinemia (increased immunoglobulin production by the spleen and bone marrow cells), and lymphoma (tumor of the lymphoid tissues).

95

Immunoglobulin G (Fc Fragment specific) Immunological Test System A Class II device that consists of the reagents used to measure, by immunochemical techniques, the Fc (carbohydrate containing) fragment of immunoglobulin G (antibodies) in urine, serum, and other biological fluids. Measurement of immunoglobulin G Fc fragments aids in the diagnosis of plasma cell antibody-forming abnormalities (e.g., gamma heavy chain disease).

Immunoglobulin G (Fd Fragment specific) Immunological Test System A Class I device that consists of the reagents used to measure, by immunochemical techniques, the amino terminal (antigen-binding) end (Fd fragment) of the heavy chain (a subunit) of the immunoglobulin antibody molecule. Measurement of immunoglobulin G Fd fragments aids in the diagnosis of plasma antibody forming cell abnormalities.

Immunoglobulin (Light chain specific) Immunological Test System A Class II device that consists of the reagents used to measure, by immunochemical techniques, both kappa and lambda types of light chain portions of immunoglobulin molecules in serum, body fluids, and tissues. In some disease states, an excess of light chains is produced by the antibody-forming cells. These free light chains, unassociated with gamma globulin molecules, can be found in a patient's body fluids and tissues. Measurements of the various amounts of the different types of light chains aid in the diagnosis of multiple myeloma (cancer of antibody-forming cells), lymphocytic neoplasms (cancer of lymphoid tissue), Waldenstrom's macroglobulinemia (increased production of large immunoglobulins), and connective tissue diseases, such as rheumatoid arthritis or systemic lupus erythematosus.

Immunoglobulins A, G, M, D, and E Immunological Test System A Class II device that consists of the reagents used to measure, by immunochemical techniques, the immunoglobulins A, G, M, D, and E (serum antibodies) in serum. Measurement of these immunoglobulins aid in the diagnosis of abnormal protein metabolism and the body's lack of ability to resist infectious agents.

Immunoreactive Insulin Test System A Class I device intended to measure immunoreactive insulin in serum and plasma. Immunoreactive insulin measurements are used in the diagnosis and treatment of various carbohydrate metabolism disorders, including diabetes mellitus, and hypoglycemia.

Impedance Phlebograph A Class II device used to provide a visual display of the venous pulse or drainage by measuring electrical impedance changes in a region of the body.

Impedance Plethysmograph A Class II device used to estimate blood flow by measuring electrical impedance changes in a region of the body.

96

Implantable Clip A clip-like Class II device intended to connect internal tissues to aid healing. It is not absorbable.

Implantable Pacemaker Pulse Generator A Class III device having a power supply and electronic circuits that produce a periodic electrical impulse to stimulate the heart. This device is used as a substitute for the heart's intrinsic pacing system to correct both intermittent and continuous cardiac rhythm disorders. This generic term includes triggered, inhibited, and asynchronous devices implanted in the human body.

Implantable Staple A staple-like Class II device intended to connect internal tissues to aid healing. It is not absorbable.

Implanted Mechanical/Hydraulic Urinary Continence Device A Class III device used to treat urinary incontinence by the application of continuous or intermittent pressure to occlude the urethra. The device may consist of implanted fixed or adjustable pressure pads or an inflatable cuff around the urethra connected to a container of radiopaque fluid implanted in the abdomen and a manual pump and valve implanted under the skin surface. The fluid is pumped from the container to inflate the cuff or pad to press on the urethra.

Impression Material (Dentistry) A Class II device composed of polymers, such as polysulfide or alginate, placed on an impression tray, to reproduce the structure and fine detail of teeth and gums. This provides models for the eventual production of restorative and prosthetic dental devices.

Impression Tube A Class I device consisting of a hollow copper tube that is used to take an impression of a single tooth. The hollow tube is filled with impression material. One end of the tube is sealed with a softened material, such as wax; the remaining end is slipped over the tooth to make an impression.

In vitro Diagnostic Products Those reagents, instruments, and systems intended for use in the diagnosis of disease or other conditions, including a determination of the state of health, in order to cure, mitigate, treat, or prevent disease or its sequelae. Such products are intended for use in the collection, preparation, and examination of specimens taken from the human body. These products are devices as defined in section 210 (h) of the Federal Food, Drug, and Cosmetic Act, and may also be biological products subject to section 351 of the Public Health Service Act (21 CFR 809.3[a], 1988).

Incentive Spirometer A Class II device that indicates the patient's breathing volume or flow. The device is used to provide an incentive to patients to improve their ventilation status.

Incubator (Neonatal) A Class II device consisting of a rigid, box-like enclosure in which an infant may be kept in a controlled environment for medical care. The device may include an AC-powered heater, a fan to circulate the warmed air, a container for water to add humidity, a control valve through which oxygen may be added, and access ports of nursing.

Incubator (Neonatal transport)   A Class II device consisting of a portable, rigid, box-like enclosure with insulated walls in which an infant may be kept in a controlled environment while being transported for medical care. The device may include straps to secure the infant, a battery-operated heater, an AC-powered battery charger, a fan to circulate the warmed air, a container for water to add humidity, and provision for a portable oxygen bottle.

Indicator Injector   A Class II device that is an electrically or gas powered device designed to inject accurately an indicator solution into the bloodstream. This device may be used in conjunction with a densitometer or thermodilution device to determine cardiac output.

Indicator (Sterilization)   A Class II device used to show, by visible or measurable evidence, that a treated medical product was sufficiently exposed to a sterilization agent to allow the user to assume that the product is sterile.

Indirect Pacemaker Generator Function Analyzer   A Class II device that is an electrically powered device used to determine pacemaker function or pacemaker battery function by periodically monitoring an implanted pacemaker pulse rate and pulse width. The device is noninvasive, and it detects pacemaker pulse rate and width via external electrodes in contact with the patient's skin.

Infant Oxygen Hood   A Class I device consisting of a rigid transparent enclosure with an open bottom placed over an infant's head. The device is connected to an external source of oxygen to maintain an oxygen-rich atmosphere for the infant.

Infant Radiant Warmer   A Class III device consisting of an infrared heating element placed over an infant to maintain the infant's body temperature by means of radiant heat. The device may contain a temperature monitoring sensor, a heat output control mechanism to regulate the infant's body temperature, and an alarm to alert operators of the device's failure. The device may be placed over a pediatric hospital bed or it may be built into the bed as a complete unit.

Infectious Mononucleosis Immunological Test System   A Class II device that consists of the reagents used to measure, by immunochemical techniques, infectious mononucleosis antibodies in serum, plasma, and body fluids. Measurements of infectious mononucleosis antibodies aid in the diagnosis of infectious mononucleosis.

Inflatable Extremity Splint   A Class I device intended to be inflated to immobilize a limb or an extremity.

Inflatable Tracheal Tube Cuff A Class II device used to provide an airtight seal between the tracheal tube and the patient's trachea.

Influenza Virus Serological Reagents Class I devices that consist of antigens and antisera and used in serological tests to identify influenza virus antibodies in a patient's serum. The identification aids in the diagnosis of influenza (flu) and provides epidemiological information on influenza. Influenza is an acute respiratory tract disease that is often epidemic.

Infrared Lamp A Class II device used to provide topical heating for therapeutic purposes by means of either a tungsten or carbon filament heated to emit a high level of incandescence (approximately 10,000 Angstroms) or a solid rod or resistance wire heated to red heat (approximately 20,000 to 40,000 Angstroms).

Injector (Gas-powered, jet) A Class II device consisting of a syringe used to administer a local anesthetic. The syringe is powered by a cartridge containing pressurized carbon dioxide that provides the pressure to force the anesthetic out of the syringe.

Injector (Nonelectrically powered fluid) A nonelectrically powered Class II device used to give a hypodermic injection by means of a narrow, high velocity jet of fluid that can penetrate the surface of the skin and deliver the fluid to the body. It may be used for mass inoculations.

Injector (Spring-powered, jet) A Class II device consisting of a syringe used to administer a local anesthetic. The syringe is powered by a spring mechanism that provides the pressure to force the anesthetic out of the syringe.

Inspiratory Airway Pressure Meter A Class II diagnostic anesthesiology device used to measure the amount of pressure produced in a patient's airway during maximal inspiration.

Instrument (Calculus removal, hand-held) A Class II hand-held metal scraper device used to remove calculus deposits from tooth surfaces.

Instrument (Dental depth gauge) A Class I device consisting of a slender metal piece that is used in endodontic (root canal) treatment to prepare for placement of a retentive or splinting pin. The device is used to measure the depth of a small hole in a tooth.

Instrument (Dental diamond) A Class II abrasive device used to smooth tooth surfaces during the fitting of crowns or bridges. The device consists of a shaft that is inserted into a handpiece and a head that has diamond chips imbedded into it. Rotation of the diamond instrument provides an abrasive action when it contacts the tooth.

Instrument (Dental hand) A Class I hand-held device used to perform various tasks in general dentistry and oral surgery procedures. The following devices are included in this generic type device: operative burnisher, operative amalgam carver, surgical bone chisel, operative amalgam and foil condenser, endodontic curette, operative curette, dental surgical elevator, operative dental excavator, operative explorer, surgical bone file, operative dental excavator, operative explorer, surgical bone file, operative margin finishing file, periodontic file, periodontic probe, surgical rongeur forceps, surgical tooth extractor instrument, operative cutting instrument, operative matrix contouring instrument, operative cutting instrument, operative margin-finishing knife, periodontic knife, periodontic marker, operative pliers, endodontic root-canal pulp-canal reamer, crown remover, periodontic scaler, collar and crown scissors, endodontic pulp canal filling material spreader, and surgical osteotome chisel.

Instrument (Dental handle)   A Class I device made of metal or plastic that is used as a grip for working tips and mirrors used during dental procedures.

Instrument (Plastic dental filling)   A Class I device made of plastic that is used to carry filling material to the site of a restoration in the oral cavity.

Interlocking Urethral Sound   A Class II device that consists of two metal sounds (elongated instruments for exploring or sounding body cavities) with interlocking ends, such as with male and female threads or a rounded point and mating socket, used in the repair of a ruptured urethra. The device may include a protective cap to fit over the metal threads.

Intermittent Pressure Measurement System   An evaluative Class II device used to measure the actual pressure between the body surface and the supporting media.

Intra-Aortic Balloon and Control System   A Class III device consisting of an inflatable balloon, which is placed in the aorta to improve cardiac function during life-threatening emergencies, and a control system for regulating the inflation and deflation of the balloon. The control system, which monitors and is synchronized with the EKG, provides a means for setting the inflation and deflation of the balloon with the cardiac cycle.

Intracardiac Patch and Pledget   A Class II device made of polypropylene, Teflon, or Dacron fabric placed in the heart and used to repair septal defects, to patch grafting, to repair tissue, and to buttress sutures.

Intracavitary Phono Catheter System   A Class II device that includes a catheter with an acoustic transducer and the associated device that processes the signal from the transducer. This device records bioacoustic phenomena from a transducer placed within the heart, blood vessels, or blood cavities.

Intraluminal Artery Stripper   A Class II device used to perform an endarterectomy (removal of plaque deposits from arteriosclerotic arteries).

Intramedullary Fixation Rod   A Class II device intended to be implanted that consists of a rod made of alloys such as cobaltchromium-molybdenum and stainless steel. It is inserted into the medullary (bone marrow) canal of long bones for the fixation of fractures.

Intraocular Fluid   A Class III device consisting of a nongaseous fluid intended to be introduced into the eye to aid performance of surgery, such as to maintain anterior chamber depth, preserve tissue integrity, protect tissue from surgical trauma, or function as a tamponade during retinal reattachment.

Intraocular Gas   A Class III device consisting of a gaseous fluid intended to be introduced into the eye to place pressure on a detached retina.

Intraocular Lens   A Class III device made of materials, such as glass or plastic, that are intended to be implanted to replace the natural lens of an eye.

Intraocular Lens Guide   A Class I device intended to be inserted into the eye during surgery to direct the insertion of an intraocular lens and to be removed after insertion is completed.

Intraocular Pressure Measuring Device   A Class III manual or ACpowered device intended to measure intraocular pressure. Also included are any devices found by FDA to be substantially equivalent to such devices. Accessories for the device may include calibrators or recorders. The device is intended for use in the diagnosis of glaucoma.

Intraoral Dental Wax   A Class I device made of wax that is used to construct patterns to customize metal dental prostheses, such as crowns and bridges. In orthodontic dentistry, the device is used to make a pattern of the patient's bite so that crowns and bridges have the proper biting surface contact.

Intraoral Source X-ray System   A Class II device that produces X-rays and is used for dental radiographic examination and diagnosis of diseases of the teeth, jaw, and oral structures. The X-ray source is located inside the mouth. This generic type of device may include patient and equipment supports and component parts.

Intraosseous Fixation Screw   A Class II metal device that is used to stabilize fractured jaw segments by inserting it into both bone segments, thereby preventing their movement.

Intraosseous Fixation Wire A Class II metal device that is used to stabilize and constrict fractured jawbone segments by wrapping the wire around the ends of the bone segments.

Intrauterine Device A Class III device placed high in the uterine fundus, with a string extending from the uterus into the vagina, that is used to prevent pregnancy. This type does not include products that function by drug activity, which are subject to the new provisions of the Federal Food, Drug, and Cosmetic Act.

Intrauterine Pressure Monitor and Accessories A Class II device designed to detect and measure intrauterine and amniotic fluid pressure with a catheter placed transcervically into the uterine cavity. The device is used to monitor the strength, duration, and frequency of uterine contractions during labor. This generic type of device includes the following accessories: signal analysis and display equipment, patient and equipment supports, and component parts.

Intravascular Administration Set A Class II device used to administer fluids from a container to the vascular system through a needle or catheter inserted into a vein. It may include tubing, flow regulator, drip chamber, and infusion line filter.

Intravascular Catheter A Class II device consisting of a slender tube constructed of metal, rubber, or plastic, that is inserted into the patient's vascular system for short-term use (fewer than thirty days) to sample blood, monitor blood pressure, or administer fluids intravenously.

Intravenous Catheter Securement Device A Class I device with an adhesive backing that is placed over a needle or catheter and is used to keep the hub of the needle or the catheter flat and securely anchored to the skin.

Introduction/Drainage Catheter and Accessories A Class I device that is a flexible single or multilumen tube intended to be used to introduce nondrug fluids into body cavities other than blood vessels, drain fluids from body cavities, or evaluate certain physiologic conditions. Examples include irrigation and drainage catheters, pediatric catheters, peritoneal catheters (including dialysis), and other general surgical catheters. An introduction/drainage catheter accessory is intended to aid in the manipulation of, or insertion of, the device into the body. Examples of accessories include adaptors, connectors, and catheter needles.

Iontophoresis Devices A Class II device used to introduce ions of soluble salts (i.e., medications) by use of a direct current into the tissues of the body for therapeutic or diagnostic purposes. An iontophoresis device for the diagnosis of cystic fibrosis is a device that induces sweating by the introduction of pilocarpine through the use of a direct current. The sweat is collected and its composition and weight are used in the diagnosis of cystic fibrosis. An iontophoresis device for dental application of fluoride is a device used to accelerate the introduction (diffusion) of fluoride ions into tooth structures to reduce hypersensitivity and for fluoride uptake in cavity prevention. An iontophoresis device for the local anesthetizing of the intact tympanic membrane is a device used to induce ions of lidocaine and epinephrine into the tympanic membrane of the ear to cause an anesthetizing effect.

Iron Binding Capacity Test System   A Class I device intended to measure iron-binding capacity in serum. Iron-binding capacity measurements are used in the diagnosis and treatment of anemia.

Iron Kinetics Test   A Class II device used to determine the plasma iron clearance and red blood cell iron incorporation. The information obtained from this system is used to diagnose iron metabolism disorders.

Iron (Nonheme) Test System   A Class I device intended to measure iron (nonheme) in serum and plasma. Iron (nonheme) measurements are used in the diagnosis and treatment of diseases such as iron deficiency anemia, hemochromatosis (a disease associated with widespread deposit in the tissues of two iron-containing pigments, hemosiderin and hemofuscin, and characterized by pigmentation of the skin), and chronic renal disease.

Irrigator (Powered nasal irrigator)   An AC-powered Class I device intended to wash the nasal cavity by means of a pressure-controlled pulsating stream of water. The device consists of a control unit and pump connected to a spray tube and nozzle.

Isocitric Dehydrogenase Test System   A Class I device intended to measure the activity of the enzyme isocitric dehydrogenase in serum and plasma. Isocitric dehydrogenase measurements are used in the diagnosis and treatment of liver disease, such as viral hepatitis, cirrhosis, or acute inflammation of the biliary tract; pulmonary disease, such as pulmonary infarction (local arrest or sudden insufficiency of the blood supply to the lungs); and diseases associated with pregnancy.

Isokinetic Testing and Evaluation System   A rehabilitative exercise Class II device used to measure, evaluate, and increase the strength of muscles and the range of motion of joints.

J

Jet Injector (Gas-powered)   A Class II device consisting of a syringe used to administer a local anesthetic. The syringe is powered by a cartridge containing pressurized carbon dioxide which provides the pressure to force the anesthetic out of the syringe.

Jet Injector (Spring-powered) A Class II device consisting of a syringe used to administer a local anesthetic. The syringe is powered by a spring mechanism which provides the pressure to force the anesthetic out of the syringe.

K

Kanamycin Test System A Class II device intended to measure kanamycin, an antibiotic drug, in plasma and serum. Measurements obtained by this device are used in the diagnosis and treatment of kanamycin overdose and in monitoring levels of kanamycin to ensure appropriate therapy.

Karaya (Denture adhesive) A Class I device composed of karaya gum (a gum from the bark of a tree of the genus *Astragalus*) that is applied to the base of a denture before the denture is inserted into the patient's mouth. The device is used to improve denture retention and comfort.

Karaya Gum with Sodium Borate Denture Adhesive A Class III device that is applied to the base of a denture before the denture is inserted into the patient's mouth. The device is used to improve denture retention and comfort. There is a lack of information concerning the safety of adhesives containing sodium borate. Sodium borate concentration of 12–20 percent of the adhesive's total weight is equivalent to 2.6–5.3 percent boron. Because at least a portion of a dental adhesive is ingested, this amount of boron could cause chronic toxicity in denture wearers.

Keratome An AC-powered or battery-powered Class I device intended to shave tissue from sections of the cornea for a lamellar (partial thickness) transplant.

Keratoprosthesis A Class III device made of plastic intended to be implanted to replace the central area of an opacified natural cornea of the eye to maintain or restore sight.

Keratoscope An AC-powered or battery-powered Class I device intended to measure and evaluate the corneal curvature of the eye. Lines and circles within the keratoscope are used to observe the corneal reflex. This generic type of device includes the photokeratoscope which records corneal curvature by taking photographs of the cornea.

Ketones (Nonquantitative) Test System A Class I device intended to identify ketones in urine and other body fluids. Identification of ketones is used in the diagnosis and treatment of acidosis (a condition characterized by abnormally high acidity of body fluids) or ketosis (a condition characterized by increased production of ketone bodies such as acetone) and for monitoring patients on ketogenic diets and patients with diabetes.

Ketosteroids Test System A 17-ketosteroids test system is a Class I device intended to measure 17-ketosteroids in urine. Measurements of 17-ketosteroids are used in the diagnosis and treatment of disorders of the adrenal cortex and gonads and of other endocrine disorders, including hypertension, diabetes, and hypothyroidism.

***Klebsiella* spp. Serological Reagents** Class I devices that consist of antigens and antisera, including antisera conjugated with a fluorescent dye (immunofluorescent reagents), that are used in serological tests to identify *Klebsiella* spp. from cultured isolates derived from clinical specimens. The identification aids in the diagnosis of infections caused by bacteria belonging to the genus *Klebsiella* and provides epidemiological information on diseases caused by *Klebsiella* spp. These organisms can cause serious urinary tract and pulmonary infections, particularly in hospitalized patients.

Knee Joint Femoral (Hemi-knee) Metallic Uncemented Prosthesis A Class III device made of alloys, such as cobalt-chromium-molybdenum, intended to be implanted to replace part of a knee joint. The device limits translation and rotation in one or more planes via the geometry of its articulating surfaces. It has no linkage across-the-joint. This generic type of device includes prostheses that consist of a femoral component with or without protuberance(s) for the enhancement of fixation and is limited to those prostheses intended for use without bone cement.

Knee Joint Femorotibial Metal/Composite Nonconstrained Cemented Prosthesis A Class II device intended to be implanted to replace part of a knee joint. The device limits minimally (less than normal anatomic constraints) translation in one or more planes. It has no linkage across-the-joint. This generic type of device includes prostheses that have a femoral condylar resurfacing component or components made of alloys, such as cobalt-chromium-molybdenum, and a tibial condylar component or components made of ultra-high molecular weight polyethylene with carbon fiber composite and are intended for use with bone cement.

Knee Joint Femorotibial Metal/Composite Semiconstrained Cemented Prosthesis A two-part Class II device intended to be implanted to replace part of a knee joint. The device limits translation and rotation in one or more planes via the geometry of its articulating surfaces. It has no linkage across-the-joint. This generic type of device includes prostheses that have a femoral component made of alloys, such as cobalt-chromium-molybdenum, and a tibial component with the articulating surfaces made of ultra-high molecular weight polyethylene with carbon fiber composite and is limited to those prostheses intended for use with bone cement.

105

Knee Joint Femorotibial Metal/Polymer Constrained Cemented Prosthesis A Class II device intended to be implanted to replace part of a knee joint. The device limits translation or rotation in one or more planes and has components that are linked together or affined. This generic type of device includes prostheses composed of a ball-and-socket joint located between a stemmed femoral and a stemmed tibial component and a runner and track joint between each pair of femoral and tibial condyles. The ball-and-socket joint is composed of a ball at the head of a column rising from the stemmed tibial component. The ball, the column, the tibial plateau, and the stem for fixation of the tibial component are made of an alloy such as cobalt-chromium-molybdenum. The ball of the tibial component is held within the socket of the femoral component by the femoral component's flat outer surface. The flat outer surface of the tibial component abuts both a reciprocal flat surface within the cavity of the femoral component and flanges on the femoral component designed to prevent distal displacement. The stem of the femoral component is made of an alloy, such as cobalt-chromium-molybdenum, but the socket of the component is made of ultra-high molecular weight polyethylene. The femoral component has metallic runners which align with the ultra-high molecular weight polyethylene tracks that press-fit into the metallic tibial component. The generic class also includes devices whose upper and lower components are linked with a solid bolt passing through a journal bearing of greater radius, permitting some rotation in the transverse plane, a minimal arc of abduction/adduction. This generic type of device is limited to those prostheses intended for use with bone cement.

Knee Joint Femorotibial Metal/Polymer Nonconstrained Cemented Prosthesis A Class II device intended to be implanted to replace part of a knee joint. The device limits minimally (less than normal anatomic constraints) translation in one or more planes. It has no linkage across-the-joint. This generic type of device includes prostheses that have a femoral condylar resurfacing component or components made of alloys, such as cobalt-chromium-molybdenum, and a tibial component or components made of ultra-high molecular weight polyethylene and are intended for use with bone cement.

Knee Joint Femorotibial Metal/Polymer Semiconstrained Cemented Prosthesis A Class II device intended to be implanted to replace part of a knee joint. The device limits translation and rotation in one or more planes via the geometry of its articulating surfaces. It has no linkage across-the-joint. This generic type of device includes prostheses that consist of a femoral component made of alloys, such as cobalt-chromium-molybdenum, and a tibial component made of ultra-high molecular weight polyethylene and is limited to those prostheses intended for use with bone cement.

106

Knee Joint Femorotibial Metallic Constrained Cemented Prosthesis A Class III device intended to be implanted to replace part of a knee joint. The device prevents dislocation in more than one anatomic plane and has components that are linked together. The only knee joint movement allowed by the device is in the sagittal plane. This generic type of device includes prostheses that have an intramedullary stem at both the proximal and distal locations. The upper and lower components may be joined either by a solid bolt or pin, an internally threaded bolt with locking screw, or a bolt retained by circlip. The components of the device are made of alloys such as cobalt-chromium-molybdenum. The stems of the device may be perforated, but are intended for use with bone cement.

Knee Joint Patellar (Hemi-knee) Metallic Resurfacing Uncemented Prosthesis A Class II or Class III device made of alloys, such as cobalt-chromium-molybdenum, intended to be implanted to replace the retropatellar articular surface of the patellofemoral joint. The device limits minimally (less than normal anatomic constraints) translation in one or more planes. It has no linkage across-the-joint. This generic type of device includes prostheses that have a retropatellar resurfacing component and an orthopedic screw to transfix the patellar remnant. This generic type of device is limited to those prostheses intended for use without bone cement. (1) Class II when intended for treatment of degenerative and posttraumatic patellar arthritis. (2) Class III when intended for uses other than treatment of degenerative and posttraumatic patellar arthritis.

Knee Joint Patellofemoral Polymer Metal Semiconstrained Cemented Prosthesis A two-part Class III device intended to be implanted to replace part of a knee joint in the treatment of primary patellofemoral arthritis or chondromalacia. The device limits translation and rotation in one or more planes via the geometry of its articulating surfaces. It has no linkage across-the-joint. This generic type of device includes a component made of alloys, such as cobalt-chromium-molybdenum or austenitic steel, for resurfacing the intercondylar groove (femoral sulcus) on the anterior aspect of the distal femur, and a patellar component made of ultra-high molecular weight polyethylene. This generic type of device is limited to those devices intended for use with bone cement. The patellar component is designed to be implanted only with its femoral component.

Knee Joint Patellofemorotibial Polymer/Metal/Metal Constrained Cemented Prosthesis A Class III device intended to be implanted to replace a knee joint. The device prevents dislocation in more than one anatomic plane and has components that are linked together. This generic type of device includes prostheses that have a femoral component, a tibial component, a cylindrical bolt and accompanying locking hardware that are all made of alloys, such as cobalt-chromium-molybdenum, and a retropatellar resurfacing component made of ultra-high molecular weight polyethylene. The retropatellar surfacing component may be attached to the resected patella either with a metallic screw or bone cement. All stemmed metallic components within this generic type are intended for use with bone cement.

Knee Joint Patellofemorotibial Polymer/Metal/Polymer Semi-constrained Cemented Prosthesis A Class II device intended to be implanted to replace a knee joint. The device limits translation and rotation in one or more planes via the geometry of its articulating surfaces. It has no linkage across-the-joint. This generic type of device includes prostheses that have a femoral component made of alloys, such as cobalt-chromium-molybdenum, and a tibial component or components and a retropatellar resurfacing component made of ultra-high molecular weight polyethylene. This generic type of device is limited to those prostheses intended for use with bone cement.

Knee Joint Tibial (Hemi-knee) Metallic Resurfacing Uncemented Prosthesis A Class II device intended to be implanted to replace part of a knee joint. The device limits minimally (less than normal anatomic constraints) translation in one or more planes. It has no linkage across-the-joint. This prosthesis is made of alloys, such as cobalt-chromium-molybdenum, and is intended to resurface one tibial condyle. The generic type of device is limited to those prostheses intended for use without bone cement.

L

Lactate Dehydrogenase Isoenzymes Test System A Class II device intended to measure the activity of lactate dehydrogenase isoenzymes (a group of enzymes with similar biological activity) in serum. Measurements of lactate dehydrogenase isoenzymes are used in the diagnosis and treatment of liver diseases, such as viral hepatitis, and myocardial infarction.

Lactate Dehydrogenase Test System A Class II device intended to measure the activity of the enzyme lactate dehydrogenase in serum. Lactate dehydrogenase measurements are used in the diagnosis and treatment of liver diseases, such as acute viral hepatitis, cirrhosis, and metastatic carcinoma of the liver; cardiac diseases, such as myocardial infarction; and tumors of the lung or kidneys.

Lactic Acid Test System A Class I device intended to measure lactic acid in whole blood and plasma. Lactic acid measurements that evaluate the acid-base status are used in the diagnosis and treatment of lactic acidosis (abnormally high acidity of the blood).

Lactic Dehydrogenase Immunological Test System A Class I device that consists of the reagents used to measure, by immunochemical techniques, the activity of the lactic dehydrogenase enzyme in serum. Increased levels of lactic dehydrogenase are found in a variety of conditions, including megaloblastic anemia (decrease in the number of mature red blood cells), myocardial infarction (heart disease), and some forms of leukemia (cancer of the blood-forming organs). However, the diagnostic usefulness of this device is limited because of the many conditions known to cause increased lactic dehydrogenase levels.

Lactoferrin Immunological Test System A Class I device that consists of the reagents used to measure, by immunochemical techniques, the lactoferrin (an iron-binding protein with the ability to inhibit the growth of bacteria in serum, human milk, body fluids and tissues). Measurement of lactoferrin may aid in the diagnosis of an inherited deficiency of this protein.

Lamp (Surgical lamp) A Class II device (including a fixture) intended to be used to provide visible illumination of the surgical field or the patient.

Lamp (Ultraviolet lamp for dermatologic disorder) A Class II device (including a fixture) intended to provide ultraviolet radiation of the body to photoactivate a drug in the treatment of a dermatologic disorder if the labelling of the drug intended for use with the device bears adequate directions for the device's use with that drug.

Lamp (Ultraviolet lamp for tanning) A Class I device (including a fixture) intended to provide ultraviolet radiation to tan the skin.

Laparoscope A Class II device used to permit direct viewing of peritoneal organs on the female genitalia. It may include trocar and cannula, scope preheater, light source, and component parts.

Laparoscopic Insufflator A Class II device used to facilitate the use of the laparoscope by filling the peritoneal cavity with gas to distend it.

Laparoscopy (Abdominoscopy, peritoneoscopy, ventroscopy) A percutaneous procedure in which an electrically lighted tubular device is inserted through the abdominal wall to visualize internal organs and structures for diagnostic or therapeutic purposes.

Lap Joint A joint made by placing one surface to be joined partly over another surface and bonding the overlapping portions.

Laryngeal Prosthesis (Taub design) A Class II device intended to direct pulmonary air flow to the pharynx in the absence of the larynx, thereby permitting esophageal speech. The device is interposed between openings in the trachea and the esophagus and may be removed and replaced each day by the patient. During phonation, air from the lungs is directed to flow through the device and over the esophageal mucosa to provide a sound source that is articulated as speech.

Laryngoscope (Flexible) A Class II device, composed of flexible fiberoptic materials, used to examine and visualize a patient's upper airway and to facilitate the placement of a tracheal tube.

Laryngoscope (Rigid) A Class II device, composed of rigid fiberoptic materials, used to examine and visualize a patient's upper airway and to facilitate the placement of a tracheal tube.

Laryngostroboscope A Class I device that is intended to allow observation of glottic action during phonation. The device operates by focusing a stroboscopic light through a lens for direct or mirror reflected viewing of glottic action. The light and microphone that amplifies acoustic signals from the glottic area may or may not contact the patient.

Laryngotracheal Topical Anesthesia Applicator A Class II device used to apply topical anesthetics to the laryngotracheal area.

Laser (Microsurgical Argon laser for all other uses) A Class III device used in laryngology and for general use in otolaryngology, that is intended to cut, destroy, or alter tissue.

Laser (Microsurgical Argon laser for use in otology) A Class II device intended to cut, destroy, or alter tissue or bone of the ear using laser light energy.

Laser Surgical Instruments for Use in General and Plastic Surgery and in Dermatology (1) A carbon dioxide laser that is a Class II device intended to cut, destroy, or remove tissue by light energy emitted by carbon dioxide. (2) An argon laser for use in dermatology that is a Class II device intended to destroy or coagulate tissue by light energy emitted by argon.

Lead Test System A Class II device intended to measure lead, a heavy metal, in blood and urine. Measurements obtained by this device are used in the diagnosis and treatment of lead poisoning.

Lead-Lined Position Indicator A Class II cone-shaped device that is attached to a dental X-ray tube and is used to aid in positioning the tube to prevent the misfocusing of the X-rays by absorbing divergent radiation, and to prevent leakage of radiation by use of the lead lining.

Lecithin/Sphingomyelin Ratio in Amniotic Fluid Test System A Class II device intended to measure the lecithin/sphingomyelin ratio in amniotic fluid. Lecithin and sphingomyelin are phospholipids (fats or fat-like substances containing phosphorus). Measurements of the lecithin/sphingomyelin ratio in amniotic fluid are used in evaluating fetal maturity.

Lectins and Proteins Lectins and protectins are proteins from plants and lower animals that cause cell agglutination in the presence of

110

certain antigens. These substances are used to detect blood group antigens for in vitro diagnostic purposes as Class II devices.

Lens Measuring Instrument   An AC-powered Class I device intended to measure the power of lenses, prisms, and their centers (e.g., lensometer).

Leptospira **spp. Serological Reagents**   Class II devices that consist of antigens and antisera used in serological tests to identify antibodies of *Leptospira* spp. in a patient's serum and/or identification of *Leptospira* spp. from cultured isolates derived from clinical specimens. Additionally, some of these antisera are conjugated with a fluorescent dye (immunofluorescent reagents) and are used to identify *Leptospira* spp. directly from clinical specimens. The identification aids in the diagnosis of leptospirosis caused by bacteria belonging to the genus *Leptospira* and provides epidemiological information on this disease. Leptospirosis infections range from mild, fever-producing illnesses to severe liver and kidney involvement producing hemorrhage and dysfunction of these organs.

Leucine Aminopeptidase Test System   A Class I device intended to measure the activity of the enzyme leucine amino-peptidase in serum, plasma, and urine. Leucine aminopeptidase measurements are used in the diagnosis and treatment of liver diseases such as viral hepatitis and obstructive jaundice.

Leukocyte Alkaline Phosphatase Test   A Class I device used to identify the enzyme leukocyte alkaline phosphatase in neutrophilic granulocytes (granular leukocytes stainable by neutral dyes). The cytochemical identification of alkaline phosphatase depends on the formation of blue granules in cells containing alkaline phosphatase. The results of this test are used to differentiate chronic granulocytic leukemia (a malignant disease characterized by excessive overgrowth of granulocytes in the bone marrow) and reactions that resemble true leukemia, such as those occurring in severe infections and polycythemia (increased total red cell mass).

Leukocyte Peroxidase Test   A Class I device used to distinguish certain myeloid cells (cells derived from the bone marrow, i.e., neutrophils, eosinophils, and monocytes) from lymphoid cells (cells of the lymphatic system) and erythroid cells (cells in the red blood cell series) on the basis of their peroxidase activity as evidenced by staining. The results of this test are used in the differential diagnosis of the leukemias.

Lidocaine Test System   A Class II device intended to measure lidocaine, an antiarrhythmic and anticonvulsant drug, in serum and plasma. Measurements obtained by this device are used in the diagnosis and treatment of lidocaine overdose or in monitoring levels of lidocaine to ensure appropriate therapy.

111

Ligator (Hemorrhoidal) A Class II device used to cut off the blood flow to hemorrhoidal tissue by means of a ligature or band placed around the hemorrhoid.

Light (Dental, operating) A Class II AC-powered device used to illuminate oral structures and operating areas.

Light (Fiberoptic, dental) A Class I AC-powered device, usually attached to a dental handpiece, that consists of glass or plastic fibers that have optical properties. The device is used to illuminate oral structures.

Light Beam Patient Position Indicator A Class II device that projects a beam of light (incoherent light or laser) to determine the alignment of the patient with a radiation beam. The beam of light is intended to be used during radiologic procedures to ensure proper positioning of the patient and to monitor alignment of the radiation beam with the patient's anatomy.

Limb Orthosis (Brace) A Class I device that is worn on the upper or lower extremities to support, to correct, or to prevent deformities or to align body structures for functional improvement. Examples of limb orthoses include the following: a whole limb and joint brace, a hand splint, an elastic stocking, a knee cage, and a corrective shoe.

Line Isolation Monitor A Class II device used to monitor the electrical leakage current from a power supply electrically isolated from the domestic power supply.

Lipase Test System A Class I device intended to measure the activity of the enzyme lipase in serum. Lipase measurements are used in diagnosis and treatment of diseases of the pancreas, such as acute pancreatitis and obstruction of the pancreatic duct.

Lipid (Total) Test System A Class I device intended to measure total lipids (fats or fat-like substances) in serum and plasma. Lipid (total) measurements are used in the diagnosis and treatment of various diseases involving lipid metabolism and atherosclerosis.

Lipoprotein Test System A Class I device intended to measure lipoprotein in serum and plasma. Lipoprotein measurements are used in the diagnosis and treatment of lipid disorders (such as diabetes mellitus), atherosclerosis, and various liver and renal diseases.

Lipoprotein X Immunological Test System A Class I device that consists of the reagents used to measure, by immunochemical techniques, lipoprotein X (a high-density lipoprotein) in serum and other body fluids. Measurement of lipoprotein X aids in the diagnosis of obstructive liver disease.

***Listeria* spp. Serological Reagents** Class I devices that consist of antigens and antisera used in serological tests to identify *Listeria* spp.

from cultured isolates derived from clinical specimens. Additionally, some of these reagents consist of Listeria spp. antisera conjugated with a fluorescent dye (immunofluorescent reagents) used to identify Listeria spp. directly from clinical specimens. The identification aids in the diagnosis of listeriosis, a disease caused by bacteria belonging to the genus Listeria, and provides epidemiological information on diseases caused by these microorganisms. Listeria monocytogenes, the most common human pathogen of this genus, causes meningitis (inflammation of the brain membranes) and meningoencephalitis (inflammation of the brain and brain membranes) and is often fatal if untreated. A second form of human listeriosis is an intrauterine infection in pregnant women that results in a high mortality rate for the infant before or after birth.

Lithium Test System A Class II device intended to measure lithium (from the drug lithium carbonate) in serum or plasma. Measurements of lithium are used to assure that the proper drug dosage is administered in the treatment of patients with mental disturbances, such as manic-depressive illness (bipolar disorder).

Lithotriptor (Electrohydraulic) A Class III AC-powered device used to fragment urinary bladder stones. It consists of a high voltage source connected by a cable to a bipolar electrode that is introduced into the urinary bladder through a cystocope. With the bladder full of water, the electrode is held against the stone and repeated electrical discharges between the two poles of the electrode cause electrohydraulic shock waves that disintegrate the stone.

Lithotriptor (Mechanical) A Class II device with steel jaws that is inserted into the urinary bladder through the urethra to grasp and crush bladder stones.

Low-Density Lipoprotein Immunological Test System A Class II device that consists of the reagents used to measure, by immunochemical techniques, the low-density lipoprotein in serum and other body fluids. Measurement of low-density lipoprotein in serum may aid in the diagnosis of disorders of lipid (fat) metabolism and help to identify young persons at risk from cardiovascular diseases.

Low-Power Binocular Loupe A Class I device that consists of two eyepieces, each with a lens or lens system, intended for medical purposes to magnify the appearance of objects.

Low-Vision Magnifier A Class I device that consists of a magnifying lens intended for use by a patient who has impaired vision. The device may be held in the hand or attached to spectacles.

Low-Vision Telescope A Class I device that consists of an arrangement of lenses or mirrors intended for use by a patient who has impaired vision to increase the apparent size of objects. This generic type of device includes hand-held or spectacle telescopes.

Luteinizing Hormone Test System   A Class I device intended to measure luteinizing hormone in serum and urine. Luteinizing hormone measurements are used in the diagnosis and treatment of gonadal dysfunction.

Lymphocyte Separation Medium   A Class I device used to isolate lymphocytes from whole blood.

Lysergic Acid Diethylamide (LDS) Test System   A Class II device intended to measure lysergic acid diethylamide, a hallucinogenic drug, in serum, urine, and gastric contents. Measurements obtained by this device are used in the diagnosis and treatment of LSD use or overdose.

Lysozyme (Muramidase) Test System   A Class I device intended to measure the activity of the bacteriolytic enzyme lysozyme (muramidase) in serum, plasma, leukocytes, and urine. Lysozyme measurements are used in the diagnosis and treatment of monocytic leukemia and kidney disease.

M

β-2-Macroglobulin Immunological Test System   A Class II device that consists of the reagents used to measure, by immunochemical techniques, the β-2-macroglobulin (a protein molecule) in serum, urine, and other body fluids. Measurement of β-2-macroglobulin aids in the diagnosis of patients with active rheumatoid arthritis and kidney disease.

Maddox Lens   A Class I device that is a series of red cylinders that change the size, shape, and color of an image. The device is intended to be hand-held or placed in a trial frame to evaluate eye muscle dysfunction.

MAF (Master files for medical devices; device master file)   To distinguish devices from drug master files (DMFs), the FDA's CDRH released a guideline for the submission of MAFs. Both filing systems use a prefix and sequential numbering to identify separate records. MAFs permit holder to: (1) Incorporate information regarding facilities, manufacturing prodecures, and controls and (2) Incorporate in a customer's application trade secret information by reference only, thereby avoiding disclosure of secrets to the customer. An MAF is reviewed only when a 510(k), IDE, or PMA application is authorized for reference. Only a detailed description of facilities, equipment, manufacturing methods, controls, specifications for in-process materials and final product constitutes a trade secret and merits this protection.

Magnesium Test System   A Class I device intended to measure

114

magnesium levels in serum and plasma. Magnesium measurements are used in the diagnosis and treatment of hypomagnesemia (abnormally low plasma levels of magnesium) and hypermagnesemia (abnormally high plasma levels of magnesium).

Magnetic Resonance Diagnostic Device A Class II device that is intended for general diagnostic use to present images that reflect the spatial distribution and/or magnetic resonance spectra which reflect frequency and distribution of nuclei exhibiting nuclear magnetic resonance. Other physical parameters derived from the images and/or spectra may also be produced. The device includes hydrogen-1 (proton) imaging, sodium-23 imaging hydrogen-1 spectroscopy, phosphorus-31 spectroscopy, and chemical shift imaging (preserving simultaneous frequency and spatial information).

Magnifying Spectacles Class I devices that consist of spectacle frames with convex lenses intended to be worn by a patient who has impaired vision to enlarge images.

Malic Dehydrogenase Test System A Class I device that is intended to measure the activity of the enzyme malic dehydrogenase in serum and plasma. Malic dehydrogenase measurements are used in the diagnosis and treatment of muscle and liver diseases, myocardial infarctions, cancer, and blood disorders, such as myelogenous (produced in the bone marrow) leukemia.

Mammographic X-ray System A Class II device intended to be used to produce radiographs of the breast. This generic type of device may include signal analysis and display equipment, patient and equipment supports, component parts, and accessories.

Mandibular Implant Facial Prosthesis A Class II device that is intended to be implanted for use in the functional reconstruction of mandibular deficits. The device is made of materials such as stainless steel, tantalum, titanium, cobalt-chromium based alloy, polytetrafluoroethylene, silicone elastomer, polyethylene, polyurethane, or polytetrafluoroethylene with carbon fiber composite.

Manometer (Venous blood pressure) A Class II device attached to a venous catheter to indicate manometrically the central or peripheral venous pressure.

Manual Adjustable Hospital Bed A Class I device consisting of a bed with a manual mechanism operated by an attendant to adjust the height and surface contour of the bed. The device includes movable and latchable side rails.

Manual Algesimeter A Class I mechanical device used to determine a patient's sensitivity to pain after using an anesthetic agent, e.g., by pricking with a sharp point.

Manual Blood Cell Counting Device A Class I device used to count red blood cells, white blood cells, and blood platelets.

Manual Cast Application and Removal Instrument A nonpowered, hand-held Class I device intended to be used in applying or removing a cast. This generic type of device includes the cast knife, cast spreader, plaster saw, plaster dispenser, and casting stand.

Manual Colony Counter A Class I device that consists of a printed grid system superimposed on an illuminated screen. Petri plates containing bacterial colonies to be counted are placed on the screen for better viewing and ease of counting. The number of colonies counted is used in the diagnosis of disease as a measure of the degree of bacterial infection.

Manual Gastroenterology-Urology Surgical Instrument and Accessories A Class I device designed to be used for gastroenterological and surgical procedures. The device may be nonpowered, hand-held, or hand manipulated. Manual instruments include the biopsy forceps cover, biopsy tray without biopsy instruments, line clamp, nonpowered rectal probe, nonelectrical clamp, needle holder, gastrourology hook, gastrourology probe and director, non-self-restraining retractor, laparotomy rings, nonelectrical snare, rectal specula, bladder neck spreader, self-retaining retractor, and scoop.

Manual Operating Table and Accessories and Manual Operating Chair and Accessories Nonpowered Class I devices, usually with movable components, intended to be used to support a patient during diagnostic examinations or surgical procedures.

Manual Ophthalmic Surgical Instrument A nonpowered, hand-held Class I device intended to aid or perform ophthalmic surgical procedures. This generic type of device includes the manual corneal bur, ophthalmic caliper, ophthalmic cannula, eyelid clamp, ophthalmic muscle clamp, iris retractor clip, orbital compressor, ophthalmic curette, cystotome, orbital depressor, lachrymal dilator, erisophake, expressor, ophthalmic forcep, ophthalmic hook, sphere introducer, ophthalmic knife, ophthalmic suturing needle, lachrymal probe, trabeculotomy probe, cornea-sclera punch, ophthalmic retractor, ophthalmic ring (Flieringa), lachrymal sac rongeur, ophthalmic scissors, enucleating snare, ophthalmic spatula, ophthalmic specula, ophthalmic spoon, ophthalmic spud, trabeculotome or ophthalmic manual trephine.

Manual Patient Rotation Bed A Class I device that turns a patient who is constrained to a reclining position. This manually operated bed is used to treat patients with severe or extensive burns or decubitus ulcers, and to aid circulation.

Manual Radionuclide Applicator System A manually operated Class I device intended to apply a radionuclide source into the body or to the surface of the body for radiation therapy. This generic type of device may include patient and equipment supports, component parts, treatment planning computer programs, and accessories.

Manual Refractor   A Class I device that is a set of lenses of various dioptric powers intended to measure the refractive error of the eye.

Manual Surgical Instrument for General Use   A nonpowered, hand-held, or hand-manipulated Class I device, either reusable or disposable, intended to be used in various general surgical procedures. The device includes the applicator, clip applier, biopsy brush, manual dermabrasion brush, scrub brush, cannula, ligature carrier, chisel, clamp, contractor, curette, cutter, dissector, elevator, skin graft expander, file, forceps, gouge, instrument guide, needle guide, hammer, hemostat, amputation hook, ligature passing and knot-tying instrument, knife, blood lancet, mallet, disposable or reusable aspiration and injection needle, disposable or reusable suturing needle, osteotome, pliers, rasp, retainer, retractor, saw, scalpel blade, scalpel handle, one-piece scalpel, snare, spatula, stapler, disposable or reusable stripper, stylet, suturing apparatus for the stomach and intestine, measuring tape, and calipers.

Manual Toothbrush   A Class I device intended to remove adherent plaque and food debris from the teeth to reduce tooth decay. It is composed of a shaft with either natural or synthetic bristles at one end.

Manufacturer   Any person, including any repacker and/or relabeller, who manufactures, fabricates, assembles, or processes a finished device. The term does not include any person who only distributes a finished device.

Manufacturing Material   Any material, such as a cleaning agent, mold-release agent, lubricating oil, or other substance, used to facilitate a manufacturing process that is not intended by the manufacturer to be included in the finished device.

Mass Spectrometer for Clinical Use   A Class I device intended to identify inorganic or organic compounds (e.g., lead, mercury, and drugs) in human specimens by ionizing the compound under investigation and separating the resulting ions by means of an electrical and magnetic field according to their mass.

Massaging Pick   A Class I pointed device made of wood or plastic that is intended to be used manually to stimulate and massage the gums to promote good periodontal condition. The end of the pick is placed at the base of the teeth and moved gently.

Master Hearing Aid   An electronic Class II device intended to simulate a hearing aid during audiometric testing. It has adjustable acoustic output levels, such as those for gain, output, and frequency response. The device is used to select and adjust a person's wearable hearing aid.

Material (Dental impression)   A Class II device composed of materials, such as alginate or polysulfide, that are placed on a preformed impression tray and used to reproduce the structure of a patient's teeth and gums. The device provides models for study and for production of restorative and prosthetic devices, such as gold inlays and dentures.

Matrix Retainer   A Class I device used to fasten together the ends of a matrix band (a mold placed around a tooth to provide support for restorative materials) and to tighten the matrix band around the tooth during restoration and filling.

Matress (Nonpowered flotation therapy)   A Class I device composed of a mattress containing air or fluid designed to support a patient and avoid excess pressure on local body areas. The device is used to treat and prevent decubitus ulcers (bedsores).

Maxwell Spot   An AC-powered Class I device that is a light source with a red and blue filter intended to test macular function.

Measuring Exercise Equipment   Manual Class II devices used to redevelop muscles, restore motion to joints, and provide general conditioning. These devices display, by means of a gauge, the amount of exercise performed. Examples of measuring exercise equipment are the therapeutic exercise bicycle, the manually propelled treadmill, and the rowing machine.

Mechanical Chair   A manually operated Class I device used to assist a disabled person in performing an activity that the person would otherwise find difficult to do or be unable to do. Examples of mechanical chairs include the following: a chair with an elevating seat used to raise a person from a sitting position to a standing position, and a chair with casters used by a person to move from one place to another while sitting.

Mechanical Denture Cleaner   A Class I AC-powered denture cleaning device that mechanically agitates the denture cleansing solution.

Mechanical Hand and Foot and Driving Controls (Automobile)   A Class II device used to enable persons who have limited use of their arms and legs to drive. This device allows the hand operation of the gas, brake, and clutch pedals, or the foot operation of the steering and gearshift.

Mechanical Lithotriptor   A Class II device with steel jaws that is inserted into the urinary bladder through the urethra to grasp and crush bladder stones.

Mechanical Table   A Class I device that has a flat surface that can be inclined or adjusted to various positions. It is used by patients with circulatory, neurological, or musculoskeletal conditions to increase tolerance to an upright or standing position.

Mechanical Walker   A four-legged Class I device used to provide moderate weight support while walking by means of a metal frame. It is used by disabled persons who lack strength, good balance, or endurance.

Mechanical Wheel Chair   A manually operated Class I device with wheels used to provide mobility to persons restricted to a sitting position.

Mediastinoscope and Accessories   A tubular, tapered, electrical endoscopic Class II device, with any of a group of accessory devices that attach to the mediastinoscope, intended to examine or treat tissue in the area separating the lungs. The device is inserted transthoracicly and is used in diagnosis of tumors and lesions and to determine whether excision of certain organs or tissues is indicated. It is typically used with a fiberoptic light source and carrier to provide illumination. The device is made of materials such as stainless steel. This generic type of device includes the flexible foreign body claw, flexible biopsy forceps, rigid biopsy curette, flexible biopsy brush, rigid biopsy forceps, and flexible biopsy curette, but excludes the fiberoptic light source and carrier.

Medical Absorbent Fiber   A Class I device made from cotton or synthetic fiber in the shape of a ball or pad used for applying medication to, or absorbing small amounts of fluids from, the patient's body surface.

Medical Cathode-Ray Tube Display   A Class II device designed primarily to display selected biological signals. This device often incorporates special display features unique to a specific biological signal.

Medical Charged-Particle Radiation Therapy System   A Class II device that produces, by acceleration, high energy charged particles (e.g., electrons and protons) intended for use in radiation therapy. This generic type of device may include signal analysis and display equipment, patient and equipment supports, treatment planning computer programs, component parts, and accessories.

Medical Device Act   The Medical Device Act, signed into law by President Gerald Ford on May 28, 1976, provided the FDA with expanded authority to regulate medical devices. Provisions of the act determine that the FDA:

- may institute regulatory action without determining that the device was in commerce
- may temporarily detain a device that is in violation of the act that presents a substantial deception or unreasonable risk of illness or injury
- may restrict the sale, distribution, or use of a device if its safety and effectiveness cannot be reasonably assured
- prescribe Good Manufacturing Practices

- require manufacturers to register and list their devices semi-annually
- classify devices into one of three categories: Class I (general controls), Class II (performance standards), and Class III (pre-market approval)
- require manufacturers of devices first marketed after May 28, 1976, to notify the agency about the safety and effectiveness of the device

Medical Device Reporting (MDR)   The MDR regulation was enacted in December 1984, and is second only to the Good Manufacturing Practice (GMP) regulation in its significance to medical device manufacturers. The regulations require manufacturers and importers to report to the FDA whenever they have reason to believe that one of their marketed devices may have caused or contributed to a death or serious injury, or malfunctioned. Under the regulation, companies have to report, irrespective of the event, whether or not the accident was the fault of the product, or even if the event was caused by product misuse. A "reportable event" must be based on information that reasonably suggests it has caused death, serious injury, or malfunction. Death is the permanent ending of all life in a person. Serious injury is an injury that (1) is life-threatening, (2) results in permanent impairment of a body function or permanent damage to body structure, or (3) necessitates medical or surgical intervention by a health-care professional to prevent permanent impairment or damage, or to relieve unanticipated temporary impairment or damage. Malfunction is a failure of the device to meet any of its performance specifications. It is reportable if the device is likely to cause or contribute to a death or serious injury if the malfunction were to occur.

Medical Gas Yoke Assembly   A Class II device used to connect medical gas cylinders to regulators and/or needle valves to supply gases for anesthesia or respiratory therapy. The device may include a gas filter.

Medical Magnetic Tape Recorder   A Class II device used to record and play back signals, from, for example, physiological amplifiers, signal conditioners, or computers.

Medical Neutron Radiation Therapy System   A Class II device intended to generate high energy neutrons for radiation therapy. This generic type of device may include signal analysis and display equipment, patient and equipment support, treatment planning computer programs, component parts, and accessories.

Medicinal Nonventilatory Nebulizer (Atomizer)   A Class I device used to deliver liquid medication to a patient in aerosol form.

Membrane Lung for Long-Term Pulmonary Support   A Class III device used to provide extracorporeal blood oxygenation for longer than twenty-four hours.

Menstrual Cup   A Class II device composed of a receptacle placed in the vagina to collect menstrual flow.

Mercury (Dental)   A Class II device composed of mercury that is used as a component of amalgam alloy in the restoration of dental cavities or broken teeth.

Mercury Alloy Dispenser   A Class I device used to measure and dispense a predetermined amount of dental mercury in droplet form and a premeasured amount of alloy pellets. The device uses a spring-activated valve to deliver the materials into a mixing capsule.

Mercury Test System   A Class I device intended to measure mercury, a heavy metal, in human specimens. Measurements obtained by this device are used in the diagnosis and treatment of mercury poisoning.

Mesh (Surgical)   A Class II device made of a metallic or polymeric screen intended to be implanted to reinforce soft tissue or bone where weakness exists. Examples of surgical mesh are metallic and polymeric mesh for hernia repair, and acetabular and cement restrictor mesh used during orthopedic surgery.

Methadone Test System   A Class II device intended to measure methadone, an addictive narcotic pain-relieving drug, in serum and urine. Measurements obtained by this device are used in the diagnosis and treatment of methadone use or overdose and to determine compliance with regulations in methadone maintenance treatment.

Methamphetamine Test System   A Class II device intended to measure methamphetamine, a central nervous system stimulating drug, in serum, plasma, and urine. Measurements obtained by this device are used in the diagnosis and treatment of methamphetamine use or overdose.

Methaqualone Test System   A Class II device intended to measure methaqualone, a hypnotic and sedative drug, in urine. Measurements obtained by this device are used in the diagnosis and treatment of methaqualone use or overdose.

Methylmalonic Acid (Nonquantitative) Test System   A Class II device intended to identify methylmalonic acid in urine. The identification of methylmalonic acid in urine is used in the diagnosis and treatment of methylmalonic aciduria, and heritable metabolic disorder, which, if untreated, may cause mental retardation.

Metreurynter-Balloon Abortion System (1156)   A Class III device used to induce abortion. The device dilates the cervix by inflating a balloon-like dilator placed in the cervical canal. This generic type of device may include pressure sources and pressure controllers.

Microbial Growth Monitor   A Class I device that measures the concentration of bacteria suspended in a liquid medium by measuring changes in light scattering properties, optical density, electrical impedance, or by making direct bacterial counts. The device aids in the diagnosis of disease.

Microbiological Assay Culture Medium   A Class I device that consists primarily of liquid and/or solid biological materials used to cultivate selected test microorganisms in order to identify and measure, by microbiological procedures, the presence and concentration of certain substances (e.g., amino acids, antimicrobial agents, vitamins) in a patient's serum. The presence and/or concentration of these substances is measured by their ability to promote or inhibit the growth of the test organism in the inoculated medium. Test results aid in the diagnosis of disease resulting from either deficient or excessive amounts of these substances in a patient's serum. Test results may also be used to monitor therapy, e.g., in the administration of certain antimicrobial drugs.

Microbiological Incubator   A Class I device with various chambers and/or water-filled compartments in which controlled environmental conditions, particularly temperature, are maintained for the cultivation of microorganisms. The device aids in the diagnosis of disease.

Microchemistry Analyzer for Clinical Use   A Class I device intended to duplicate manual analytical procedures by performing automatically various steps, such as pipetting, preparing filtrates, heating, and measuring color intensity. The distinguishing characteristic of the device is that it requires only microvolume samples obtainable from pediatric patients. This device is intended for use in conjunction with certain materials to measure a variety of analytes.

Microorganism Differentiation and Identification Device   A Class I device that consists of one or more components (e.g., differential culture media, biochemical reagents, and/or paper disks or paper strips impregnated with test reagents) that are usually contained in individual compartments and that are used to differentiate and identify selected microorganisms or groups of microorganisms. The device aids in the diagnosis of disease.

Microscope and Accessories   Class I optical devices used to enlarge images of specimens, preparations, and cultures for examination. Variations of microscopes and accessories (through a change in light source) used in clinical laboratories include the following: (1) Phase contrast microscopes that permit visualization of unstained preparations by altering the phase relationship of light that passes around the object and through the object. (2) Fluorescence microscopes that permit examination of specimens stained with fluorochromes that fluoresce under ultraviolet light. (3) Inverted stage microscopes that permit examination of tissue cultures or other biological specimens in bottles or tubes with the light source mounted above the specimens.

Microsedimentation Centrifuge A Class I device used to sediment red blood cells for the microsedimentation rate test.

Microsurgical Argon Laser for All Other Uses A Class III device (including use in laryngology and for general use in otolaryngology) that is intended to cut, destroy, or alter tissue.

Microsurgical Argon Laser for Use in Otology A Class II device intended to cut, destroy, or alter tissue or bone of the ear using laser light energy.

Microtiter Diluting and Dispensing Device A Class I mechanical device used to dispense and/or serially dilute biological or chemical reagents in very small quantities for use in a variety of diagnostic procedures.

Microtitrator for Clinical Use A Class I device intended for use in microanalysis to measure the concentration of a substance by reacting it with a measured microvolume of a known standardized solution.

Microwave Diathermy A Class II device for use in applying therapeutic deep heat that applies high-frequency energy at microwave frequencies (915 megahertz to 2450 megahertz) to specific areas of the body. Such tissue heating is used as adjunctive therapy for the relief of pain in medical conditions such as muscle spasms and joint contractures.

Middle Ear Mold A preformed Class II device that is intended to be implanted to reconstruct the middle ear cavity during repair of the tympanic membrane. The device permits an ample, air-filled cavity to be maintained in the middle ear and promotes regeneration of the mucous membrane lining of the middle ear cavity. A middle ear mold is made of materials such as polyamide, polytetrafluoroethylene, silicone elastomer, or polyethylene, but does not contain porous polyethylene.

Miniature Pressure Transducer A Class II device used to measure the pressure between a device and soft tissue by converting mechanical inputs to analog electrical signals.

Mobile X-ray System A transportable Class II device system intended to be used to generate and control X-ray for diagnostic procedures. This generic type of device may include signal analysis and display equipment, patient and equipment supports, component parts, and accessories.

Moist Heat Pack A Class I device consisting of silica gel in a fabric container used to retain an elevated temperature for moist heat therapy.

Moist Steam Cabinet A Class II device that delivers a flow of heated, moisturized air to a patient in an enclosed unit to treat arthritis and fibrosis (a formation of fibrous tissue) and to increase local blood flow.

Monitor (Airway pressure)   A Class II device used to measure upper airway pressure. The device may include a pressure gauge and an alarm.

Monitor (Breathing frequency)   A Class II device used to measure a patient's respiratory rate. The device provides an audible or visible alarm when the respiratory rate is outside predetermined limits.

Monitor (Cutaneous oxygen)   A Class II device used to monitor relative changes in the cutaneous oxygen tension by using a non-invasive sensor (e.g., Clark-type polarographic electrode) placed on the patient's skin.

Monitor (Lung water)   A Class III device used to monitor the trend of fluid volume changes in a patient's lung by measuring changes in thoracic electrical impedance by means of electrodes placed on the chest.

Monitor (Ultrasonic air embolism)   A Class II device used to detect air bubbles in a patient's bloodstream. It may use Doppler or other ultrasonic principle.

Morphine Test System   A Class II device intended to measure morphine, an addictive, narcotic pain-relieving drug, and its analogs in serum, urine, and gastric contents. Measurements obtained by this device are used in the diagnosis and treatment of morphine use of overdose and in monitoring levels of morphine and its analogs to ensure appropriate therapy.

Motorized Three-Wheeled Vehicle   A gasoline-fueled or battery-powered Class II device that is used for outside transportation by disabled persons.

Mouth Mirror   A Class I hand-held or glass device that is used as a visual aid to reflect oral structures during examination and treatment of the teeth and the oral cavity.

Mucopolysaccharides (Nonquantitative) Test System   A Class I device intended to measure the levels of mucopolysaccharides in urine. Mucopolysaccharide measurements in urine are used in the diagnosis and treatment of various inheritable disorders that affect bone and connective tissues, such as Hurler's, Hunter's, Sanfilippo's, Scheie's, Morquio's, and Maroteaux-Lamy syndromes.

Multifunction Physical Therapy Table   A Class II device consisting of a motorized table equipped to provide patients with heat, traction, and muscle relaxation therapy.

Multiple Autoantibodies Immunological Test System   A Class II device that consists of the reagents used to measure, by immunochemical techniques, the autoantibodies (antibodies pro-

124

duced against the body's own tissues) in human serum and other biological fluids. Measurement of multiple autoantibodies aids in the diagnosis of autoimmune disorders (diseases produced when the body's own tissues are injured by autoantibodies). The device aids in the evaluation of patients in whom systemic lupus erythematosus (a multisystem autoimmune disease) or one of several other autoimmune connective tissue diseases produces a spectrum of autoantibodies (antibodies produced against patient's own tissues) against a variety of tissues. These multiple antibodies are not specific and will react with the antigenic components of cells from many species. Multiple autoantibodies may belong to any of the immunoglobulin classes (IgA, IgD, IgE, IgG, and IgM). Immunological procedures that have been used to detect multiple autoantibodies include: complement fixation, passive hemagglutination, passive agglutination, gel diffusion, counter immunoelectrophoresis, radioimmunoassay, and immunofluorescence assays. A significant number of apparently normal individuals also demonstrate autoantibodies in their serum. Consequently, for the definite diagnosis of a given autoimmune disorder, additional immunological tests are needed to interpret the significance of detecting multiple autoantibodies in serum.

Multipurpose Culture Medium A Class I device that consists primarily of liquid and/or solid biological materials used for the cultivation and identification of several types of microorganisms without the need of additional nutritional supplements. Test results aid in the diagnosis of disease and also provide epidemiological information on diseases caused by these microorganisms.

Multipurpose System for in vitro Coagulation Studies A Class II device consisting of one automated or semiautomated instrument and its associated reagents and controls. This system is used to perform a series of coagulation studies and coagulation factor assays.

Mumps Virus Serological Reagents Class I devices that consist of antigens and antisera used in serological tests to identify mumps virus antibodies in a patient's serum. Additionally, some of these reagents consist of antisera conjugated with a fluorescent dye (immunofluorescent reagents) used in serological tests to identify mumps viruses from tissue culture isolates derived from clinical specimens. The identification aids in the diagnosis of mumps and provides epidemiological information on mumps. Mumps is an acute contagious disease, particularly in children, characterized by an enlargement of one or both of the parotid glands (glands situated near the ear), although other organs may also be involved.

***Mycobacterium tuberculosis* Immunofluorescent Reagent** Class I devices that consist of antisera conjugated with a fluorescent dye used to identify *Mycobacterium tuberculosis* directly from clinical specimens. The identification aids in the diagnosis of tuberculosis and provides epidemiological information on this disease.

Mycobacterium tuberculosis is the common causative organism in human tuberculosis, a chronic infectious disease characterized by formation of tubercles (small rounded nodules) and tissue necrosis (destruction), usually occurring in the lung.

Mycoplasma Detection Media and Components   Class I products that are used to detect and isolate mycoplasma pleuropneumonia-like organisms (PPLO), a common microbial contaminant in cell cultures.

***Mycoplasma* spp. Serological Reagents**   Class I devices that consist of antigens and antisera used as serological tests to identify *Mycoplasma* spp. antibodies in a patient's serum. Additionally, some of these reagents consist of *Mycoplasma* spp. antisera conjugated with a fluorescent dye (immunofluorescent reagents) used to identify *Mycoplasma* spp. directly from clinical specimens. The identification aids in the diagnosis of disease caused by bacteria belonging to the genus *Mycoplasma* and provides epidemiological information on diseases caused by these microorganisms. *Mycoplasma* spp. are associated with inflammatory conditions of the urinary and respiratory tracts, the genitals, and the mouth. The effects in humans of infection with *Mycoplasma pneumoniae* range from inapparent infection to mild or severe upper respiratory disease, ear infection, and bronchial pneumonia.

Myoglobin Immunological Test System   A Class I device that consists of the reagents used to measure, by immunochemical techniques, the myoglobin (an oxygen storage protein found in muscle) in serum and other body fluids. Measurement of myoglobin aids in the rapid diagnosis of patients with renal or heart disease.

N

Nasal Oxygen Cannula   A Class I device composed of a two-pronged cannula used to administer oxygen to a patient through the nose.

Nasal Oxygen Catheter   A Class I device that is inserted through a patient's nostril to administer oxygen.

Nasogastric Tube (Feeding tube; Levine tube)   A Class I device inserted through the nose into the upper gastrointestinal tract to provide alimentation, or to remove air or liquid.

Nasolaryngoscope (Flexible or rigid) and Accessories   A tubular endoscopic device with any of a group of accessory Class II devices that attach to the nasopharyngoscope and is intended to examine or treat the nasal cavity and nasal pharynx. It is typically used with a fiberoptic light source and carrier to provide illumination. The device is made of materials such as stainless steel and flexible plastic. This generic type of device includes the antroscope, nasopharyngolaryngoscope, nasosinuscope, nasoscope, postrhinoscope, rhinoscope, salpingoscope, flexible foreign body claw, flexible biopsy forceps, rigid biopsy curette, flexible biopsy brush, rigid biopsy forceps and flexible biopsy curette, but excludes the fiberoptic light source and carrier.

Nasopharyngeal Catheter A device consisting of a bougie or filiform catheter that is intended for use in probing or dilating the eustachian tube. This generic type of device includes eustachian catheters.

Nd:YAG Laser for Posterior Capsulotomy A Class II device consisting of a mode-locked or Q-switched, solid state Nd:YAG laser intended for posterior capsulotomy, that generates short pulse, low energy, high power, coherent optical radiation. When the laser output is combined with focusing optics, the high irradiance at the target causes tissue disruption via optical breakdown. A visible aiming system is utilized to target the invisible Nd:YAG laser radiation on or in close proximity to the target tissue.

Nearpoint Ruler A Class I device calibrated in centimeters intended to measure the nearpoint of convergence (the point to which the visual lines are directed when convergence is at its maximum).

Nebulizer A Class II device used to add particulate liquids via a spray to inspired gases that are directly delivered to the airways. Included are: gas, heater, venturi, and refillable nebulizers.

Needle (Dental injecting) A Class II slender, hollow metal device with a sharp point that is attached to a syringe and is used to inject anesthetics and other drugs.

Needle-Type Epilator A Class II device intended to destroy the dermal papilla of a hair by applying electric current at the tip of a fine needle that has been inserted close to the hair shaft, under the skin, and into the dermal papilla. The electric current may be high-frequency AC current, high-frequency AC combined with DC current, or DC current only.

***Neisseria* spp. Direct Serological Test Reagents** Class II devices that consist of antigens and antisera used in serological tests to identify *Neisseria* spp. from cultured isolates derived from clinical specimens. Additionally, some of these reagents consist of *Neisseria* spp. antisera conjugated with a fluorescent dye (immunofluorescent reagents) which may be used to detect the presence of *Neisseria* spp. directly from clinical specimens. The identification aids in the diagnosis of disease caused by bacteria belonging to the genus *Neisseria*, such as epidemic cerebrospinal meningitis, meningococcal disease, and gonorrhea, a venereal disease, and also provides epidemiological information on diseases caused by these microorganisms. The device does not include products for the detection of gonorrhea in humans by indirect methods, such as detection of antibodies or of oxidase produced by gonococcal organisms.

Neon Gas Analyzer A Class II diagnostic anesthesiology device used to measure the concentration of neon in a gas mixture. The device may use analytical techniques, such as thermal conductivity or mass spectrometry.

Neonatal Eye Pad An opaque Class I device used to cover and protect the eye of an infant during therapeutic procedures, such as phototherapy.

Neonatal Incubator A Class II device consisting of a rigid, box-like enclosure in which an infant may be kept in a controlled environment for medical care. The device may include an AC-powered heater, a fan to circulate the warmed air, a container for water to add humidity, a control valve through which oxygen may be added, and access ports of nursing.

Neonatal Transport Incubator A Class II device consisting of a portable, rigid, box-like enclosure with insulated walls in which an infant may be kept in a controlled environment while being transported for medical care. The device may include straps to secure the infant, a battery-operated heater, an AC-powered battery charger, a fan to circulate the warmed air, a container for water to add humidity, and provision for a portable oxygen bottle.

Nephelometer for Clinical Use A Class I device intended to estimate the concentrate of particles in a suspension by measuring their light-scattering properties (the deflection of light rays by opaque particles in their path). The device is used in conjunction with certain materials to measure the concentration of a variety of analytes.

Nerve Stimulator A Class II device used to electrically stimulate a peripheral nerve to relieve severe intractable pain. It consists of an implanted receiver with electrodes placed around a peripheral nerve and an external transmitter for transmitting the stimulating pulses across the skin to the implanted receiver.

Neuroleptic Drugs Radioreceptor Assay Test System A Class II device intended to measure in serum or plasma, the dopamine receptor blocking activity of neuroleptic drugs and their active metabolites. A neuroleptic drug has antipsychotic action affecting principally psychomotor activity, is generally without hypnotic effects, and is a tranquilizer. Measurements obtained by this device are used to aid in determining whether a patient is taking the prescribed dosage level of such drugs.

Nitrite (Nonquantitative) Test System A Class I device intended to identify nitrite in urine. Nitrite identification is used in the diagnosis and treatment of urinary tract infection of bacterial origin.

Nitrogen Gas Analyzer   A Class II diagnostic anesthesiology device used to measure the concentration of nitrogen in a gas mixture. The device may use analytical techniques, such as gas chromatography or mass spectrometry.

Nitrogen (Amino-nitrogen) Test System   A Class I device intended to measure amino acid nitrogen levels in serum, plasma, and urine. Nitrogen (amino-nitrogen) measurements are used in the diagnosis and treatment of certain forms of severe liver disease and renal disorders.

Nonabsorbable Gauze for Internal Use   A Class II device made of an open mesh fabric intended to be used inside the body or a surgical incision or applied to internal organs or structures to control bleeding, absorb fluid, or protect organs or structures from abrasion, drying, or contamination. The device is woven from material made of not less than 50 percent, by mass, cotton, cellulose, or a simple chemical derivative of cellulose, and contains X-ray detectable elements.

Nonabsorbable Polyamide Surgical Suture   A sterile Class II device made of a flexible thread prepared from long-chain aliphatic polymers Nylon 6 and Nylon 6,6 and is indicated for use in soft tissue approximation. The polyamide surgical suture meets *United States Pharmacopeia* (U.S.P.) requirements as described in the U.S.P. *Monograph for Nonabsorbable Surgical Sutures.* It may be monofilament or multifilament in form, uncoated or coated, and undyed or dyed with an appropriate FDA-listed color additive. Also, the suture may be provided with or without a standard needle attached.

Nonabsorbable Poly(ethylene terephthalate) Surgical Suture   A Class II multifilament, nonabsorbable, sterile, flexible thread device prepared from fibers of high molecular weight, long-chain, linear polyesters having recurrent aromatic rings as an integral component and is indicated for use in soft tissue approximation. The poly(ethylene terephthalate) surgical suture meets U.S.P. requirements as described in the U.S.P. *Monograph for Nonabsorbable Surgical Sutures.* It may be provided uncoated or coated, and undyed or dyed with an appropriate FDA-listed color additive. Also, the suture may be provided with or without a standard needle attached.

Nonbreathing Mask   A Class II device fitting over the face used to supplement a patient's inspired oxygen. It uses one-way valves to prevent the patient from rebreathing exhaled gases.

Nonbreathing Valve   A Class II device consisting of a one-way valve that directs inspiratory gas flow to the patient and exhaled gases into the atmosphere.

Nonelectrically Powered Fluid Injector   A nonelectrically powered Class II device used to give a hypodermic injection by means of a narrow, high velocity jet of fluid which can penetrate the surface of the skin and deliver the fluid to the body. It may be used for mass inoculations.

Nonfetal Ultrasonic Monitor A Class II device that projects a continuous high-frequency sound wave into body tissue other than a fetus to determine frequency changes (Doppler shift) in the reflected wave and is intended for use in the investigation of nonfetal blood flow and other nonfetal body tissues in motion. This generic type of device may include signal analysis and display equipment, patient and equipment supports, component parts, and accessories.

Nonimage Intensified Fluoroscopic X-ray System A Class II device intended to be used to visualize anatomical structures by using a fluorescent screen to convert a pattern of X-radiation into a visible image. This generic type of device may include signal analysis and display equipment, patient and equipment supports, component parts, and accessories.

Nonimplanted Electrical Continence Device A Class III device that consists of a pair of electrodes on a plug or a pessary that are connected by an electrical cable to a battery-powered pulse source. The plug or pessary is inserted into the rectum or into the vagina and is used to stimulate the muscles of the pelvic floor to maintain urinary or fecal continence. When necessary, the plug or pessary may be removed by the user.

Noninflatable Extremity Splint A Class I device intended to immobilize a limb or an extremity. It is not inflatable.

Noninvasive Traction Component A Class I device, such as a head halter, pelvic belt, or a traction splint, that does not penetrate the skin and is intended to assist in connecting a patient to a traction apparatus so that a therapeutic pulling force may be applied to the patient's body.

Nonmeasuring Exercise Equipment Class I devices used to redevelop muscles, restore motion to joints, and provide general physical conditioning. Examples of nonmeasuring exercise equipment are prone scooter boards, parallel bars, mechanical treadmills, and exercise tables.

Nonpneumatic Tourniquet A Class I device consisting of a strap or tubing intended to be wrapped around a patient's limb and tightened to reduce circulation.

Nonpowered Breast Pump A Class I manual suction device used for postpartum extraction of milk from the breast.

Nonpowered Communication System A Class I mechanical device used to assist a patient in communicating when physical impairment prevents writing, telephone use, reading, or talking. Examples of nonpowered communications systems include the following: an alphabet board, a telephone holder, and a page turner.

Nonpowered Dynamometer A mechanical Class I device intended for medical purposes to measure the pinch and grip muscle strength of a patient's hand.

Nonpowered Flotation Therapy Mattress A Class I device composed of a mattress, containing air or fluid, designed to support a patient and avoid excess pressure on local body areas. The device is used to treat and prevent decubitus ulcers (bedsores).

Nonpowerd Goniometer A mechanical Class I device intended for medical purposes to measure the range of motion of joints.

Nonpowered Orthopedic Traction Apparatus and Accessories A Class I device that consists of a rigid frame with nonpowered traction accessories, such as cords, pulleys, or weights, and that is intended to apply a therapeutic pulling force to the skeletal system.

Nonpowered Sitz Bath A Class I device composed of a tub to be filled with water that is used in external hydrotherapy to relieve pain or pruritis and to accelerate the healing of inflamed or traumatized tissues of the perianal and perineal areas.

Nonpowered, Single Patient, Portable Suction Apparatus A Class I device that consists of a manually operated, plastic, disposable evacuation system intended to provide a vacuum for suction drainage of surgical wounds.

Nonroller-Type Cardiopulmonary Bypass Blood Pump A Class III device that uses a method other than revolving rollers to pump the blood through the cardiopulmonary bypass circuit during bypass surgery.

Nose Clip A Class I device used to close the external nares during diagnostic or therapeutic procedures.

Nose Prosthesis A silicone rubber, solid, Class II device intended to be implanted to augment or reconstruct the nasal dorsum.

Nuclear Anthropomorphic Phantom A human tissue facsimile Class I device that contains a radioactive source or a cavity in which a radioactive sample can be inserted. It is intended to calibrate nuclear uptake probes or other medical instruments.

Nuclear Electrocardiograph Synchronizer A Class I device intended for use in nuclear radiology to relate the time of image formation to the cardiac cycle during the production of dynamic cardiac images.

Nuclear Flood Source Phantom A Class I device that consists of a radioluscent container filled with a uniformly distributed solution of a desired radionuclide. It is intended to calibrate a medical gamma camera-collimator system for uniformity of response.

Nuclear Rectilinear Scanner   A Class I device intended to image the distribution of radionuclides in the body by means of a detector (or detectors) whose position moves in two directions with respect to the patient. This generic type of device may include signal analysis and display equipment, patient and equipment supports, radionuclide anatomical markers, component parts, and accessories.

Nuclear Scanning Bed   A Class I device composed of an adjustable bed intended to support a patient during a nuclear medicine procedure.

Nuclear Sealed Calibration Source   A Class I device that consists of an encapsulated reference radionuclide intended for calibration of medical nuclear radiation detectors.

Nuclear Tomography System   A Class II device intended to detect nuclear radiation in the body and produce images of a specific cross-sectional plane of the body by blurring or eliminating detail from other planes. This generic type of devices may include signal analysis and display equipment, patient and equipment supports, radionuclide anatomical markers, component parts, and accessories.

Nuclear Uptake Probe   A Class I device intended to measure the amount of radionuclide taken up by a particular organ or body region. This generic type of device may include a single or multiple detector probe, signal analysis and display equipment, patient and equipment supports, component parts, and accessories.

Nuclear Whole Body Counter   A Class I device intended to measure the amount of radionuclides in the entire body. This generic type of device may include signal analysis and display equipment, patient and equipment supports, component parts, and accessories.

Nuclear Whole Body Scanner   A Class I device intended to measure and image the distribution of radionuclides in the body by means of a wide-aperture detector whose position moves in one direction with respect to the patient. This generic type of device may include signal analysis and display equipment, patient and equipment supports, radionuclide anatomical markers, component parts, and accessories.

5′-Nucleotidase Test System   A Class I device intended to measure the activity of the enzyme 5′-nucleotidase in serum and plasma. Measurements of 5′-nucleotidase are used in the diagnosis and treatment of liver diseases and in the differentiation between liver and bone diseases in the presence of elevated serum alkaline phosphatase activity.

Nystagmus Tape   A Class I device that is a long, narrow strip of fabric or other flexible material on which a series of objects are printed.

The device is intended to be moved across a patient's field of vision to elicit optokinetic nystagmus (abnormal and irregular eye movements) and to test for blindness.

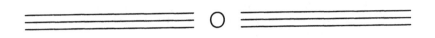

Obstetric Anesthesia Set An assembly of Class II antiseptic solution, needles, needle guides, syringes, and other accessories, intended for use with an anesthetic drug. This device is used to administer regional blocks (e.g., paracervical, uterosacral, and pudendal), that may be used during labor, delivery, or both. Included in this generic type of device are those devices identified as "paracervical anesthesia set" and "pudendal anesthesia set."

Obstetric Data Analyzer A Class III device used to interpret fetal status during labor and to warn of possible fetal distress by analyzing electronic signal data obtained from fetal or maternal electronic or other monitors. This generic type of device includes signal analysis and display equipment, electronic interfaces for other equipment, and power supplies and component parts.

Obstetric Fetal Destructive Instrument A Class II device designed to crush or pull the fetal body to facilitate the delivery of a dead or anomalous (abnormal) fetus. Included in this generic type of device are those devices identified as "cleidoclast," "cranioclast," "craniotribe," and "destructive hook."

Obstetric Forceps A Class II device with two blades and handles. It is intended to grasp and apply traction to the fetal head in the birth passage and facilitate delivery.

Obstetric Table and Accessories A Class II device with adjustable sections used to support a patient in the various positions required during obstetric and gynecologic procedures. This generic type of device may include the following accessories: patient equipment, support attachments, and cabinets for warming instruments and disposing of wastes. Included in this generic type are those devices identified as "AC-powered obstetric table and accessories," "manual obstetric table and accessories," and "lithotomy drape clip."

Obstetric Ultrasonic Transducer and Accessories A Class II device used to apply ultrasonic energy to, and receive ultrasonic energy from, the body in conjunction with an obstetric monitor or imager. The device converts electrical signals into ultrasonic energy, and vice versa, by means of an assembly distinct from an ultrasonic generator. This generic type of device includes the following accessories: coupling gel, preamplifiers, amplifiers, signal conditioners with their power supply, connecting cables, and component parts. This generic type of device does not include devices used to generate the ultrasonic frequency electrical signals for application.

Obstetric-Gynecologic General Manual Instrument   One of a group of Class I devices used to perform simple obstetric and gynecologic manipulative functions. This generic type of device consists of the following: (1) Episiotomy scissors—a cutting instrument with two opposed shearing blades used for surgical incision of the vulvar orifice for obstetrical purposes. (2) Fiberoptic metal vaginal speculum—a metal instrument, with fiberoptic light, used to expose the interior of the vagina. (3) Metal vaginal speculum—a metal instrument used to expose the interior of the vagina. (4) Umbilical scissors—a cutting instrument with two opposed shearing blades used to cut the umbilical cord. (5) Uterine clamp—an instrument used to effect the compression of the uterus. (6) Uterine packer—an instrument used to introduce dressings into the uterus or vagina. (7) Vaginal applicator—an instrument used to insert medication into the vagina. (8) Vaginal retractor—an instrument used to maintain vaginal exposure by separating the edges of the vagina and holding back the tissue. (9) Gynecological fibroid hook—an instrument used to exert traction upon a fibroid. (10) Pelvimeter (external)—an instrument used to measure the external diameters of the pelvis.

Obstetric-Gynecologic Specialized Manual Instrument   One of a group of Class II devices used during obstetric-gynecologic procedures to perform manipulative diagnostic and surgical functions (e.g., dilating, grasping, measuring, and scraping) where structural integrity is the chief criterion of device performance. This type of device consists of the following: (1) Amniotome—an instrument used to rupture the fetal membranes. (2) Circumcision clamp—an instrument used to compress the foreskin of the penis during circumcision of a male infant. (3) Umbilical clamp—an instrument used to compress the umbilical cord. (4) Uterine curette—an instrument used to scrape and remove material from the uterus. (5) Fixed-sized cervical dilator—any of a series of bougies of various sizes used to enlarge the cervix by stretching. (6) Uterine elevator—an instrument inserted into the uterus used to lift and manipulate the uterus. (7) Gynecological surgical forceps—an instrument with two blades and handles used to pull, grasp, or compress during gynecological examination. (8) Cervical cone knife—a cutting instrument used to excise and remove tissue from the cervix. (9) Gynecological cerclage needle—a sharp, loop-like instrument used to suture. (10) Hook-type contraceptive intrauterine device (IUD) remover—an instrument used to remove an IUD from the uterus. (11) Gynecological fibroid screw—an instrument used to hold onto a fibroid. (12) Uterine sound—an instrument used to determine the depth of the uterus. (13) Cytological cervical spatula—a blunt instrument used to scrape and remove cytological material from the surface of the cervix or vagina. (14) Gynecological biopsy forceps—an instrument with two blades and handles used for gynecological biopsy procedures. (15) Uterine tenaculum—a hook-like instrument used to seize and hold the cervix or fundus. (16) Internal pelvimeter—an instrument used to measure the diameter and capacity of the pelvis within the vagina. (17) Nonmetal vaginal speculum—a nonmetal instrument used to expose the interior of the vagina. (18) Fiberoptic nonmetal vaginal speculum—a nonmetal instrument, with fiberoptic light, used to expose the interior of the vagina.

Obstetric-Gynecologic Ultrasonic Imager A Class II device designed to transmit and receive ultrasonic energy into and from a female patient by pulsed echoscopy. This device is used to provide a visual representation of some physiological or artificial structure, or of a fetus, for diagnostic purposes during a limited period of time. This generic type of device may include signal analysis and display equipment, electronic interfaces for other equipment, patient and equipment supports, coupling gel, and component parts. This generic type of device does not include devices used to monitor the changes in some physiological condition over long periods of time.

Occult Blood Test A Class II device used to detect occult blood in urine or feces. (Occult blood is blood present in small quantities and is detectable only by chemical, microscopic, or spectroscopic tests.)

Ocular Esthesiometer A Class I device, such as a single-hair brush, intended to touch the cornea to assess corneal sensitivity.

Ocular Pressure Applicator A manual Class II device consisting of a sphygmomanometer-type squeeze bulb, a dial indicator, a band, and bellows, that is intended to apply pressure on the eye in preparation for ophthalmic surgery.

Ocular Surgery Irrigation Device A Class I device intended to be suspended over the ocular area during ophthalmic surgery to deliver continuous, controlled irrigation to the surgical field.

Operating Headlamp An AC-powered or battery-powered Class I device intended to be worn on the user's head to provide a light source to aid visualization during surgical, diagnostic, or therapeutic procedures.

Operating Tables and Accessories and Operating Chairs and Accessories AC-powered or air-powered Class I devices, usually with movable components, intended for use during diagnostic examinations or surgical procedures to support and position a patient.

Ophthalmic Bar Prism A Class I device that is a bar composed of fused prisms of gradually increasing strengths intended to measure latent and manifest strabismus (eye muscle deviation) or the power of fusion of a patient's eyes.

Ophthalmic Bar Reader A Class I device that consists of a magnifying lens intended for use by a patient who has impaired vision. The device is placed directly onto reading material to magnify print.

Ophthalmic Beta Radiation Source A Class II device intended to apply superficial radiation to benign and malignant ocular growths.

Ophthalmic Camera An AC-powered Class II device intended to take photographs of the eye and the surrounding area.

Ophthalmic Chair An AC-powered or manual Class I device with adjustable positioning in which a patient is to sit or recline during ophthalmological examination or treatment.

Ophthalmic Conformer A Class II device, usually made of molded plastic, intended to be inserted temporarily between the eyeball and eyelid to maintain space in the orbital cavity and prevent closure or adhesions during the healing process following surgery.

Ophthalmic Contact Lens Radius Measuring Device An AC-powered Class I device that is a microscope and dial gauge intended to measure the radius of a contact lens.

Ophthalmic Electrolysis Unit An AC-powered or battery-powered device intended to destroy ocular hair follicles by applying a galvanic electrical current. Class I for the battery-powered device. Class II for the AC-powered device.

Ophthalmic Eye Shield A Class I device that consists of a plastic or aluminum eye covering intended to protect the eye or retain dressing materials in place.

Ophthalmic Fresnel Prism A Class I device that is a thin plastic sheet with embossed rulings that provides the optical effect of a prism. The device is intended to be applied to spectacle lenses to give a prismatic effect.

Ophthalmic Instrument Stand An AC-powered or nonpowered Class I device intended to store ophthalmic instruments in a readily accessible position.

Ophthalmic Instrument Table An AC-powered or manual Class I device on which ophthalmic instruments are intended to be placed.

Ophthalmic Isotope Uptake Probe An AC-powered Class II device intended to measure, by a probe which is placed in close proximity to the eye, the uptake of a radioisotope (phosphorus 32) by tumors to detect tumor masses on, around, or within the eye.

Ophthalmic Knife Test Drum A Class I device intended to test the keenness of ophthalmic surgical knives to determine whether resharpening is needed.

Ophthalmic Laser An AC-powered Class II device intended to coagulate or cut tissue of the eye, orbit, or surrounding skin by a laser beam.

Ophthalmic Lens Gauge   A calibrated Class I device intended to manually measure the curvature of a spectacle lens.

Ophthalmic Operating Spectacles (Loupes)   Class I devices that consist of convex lenses or lens systems intended to be worn by a surgeon to magnify the surgical site during ophthalmic surgery.

Ophthalmic Photocoagulator   An AC-powered Class II device intended to use the energy from an extended noncoherent light source to occlude blood vessels of the retina, choroid, or iris.

Ophthalmic Preamplifier   An AC-powered or battery-powered Class II device intended to amplify electrical signals from the eye in electroretinography (recording retinal action currents from the surface of the eyeball after stimulation by light), electrooculography (testing for retinal dysfunction by comparing the standing potential in the front and the back of the eyeball), and electromyography (recording electrical currents generated in active muscle).

Ophthalmic Prism Reader   A Class I device intended for use by a patient who is in a supine position to change the angle of print to aid reading.

Ophthalmic Projector   An AC-powered Class I device intended to project an image on a screen for vision testing.

Ophthalmic Refractometer   An automatic AC-powered Class II device that consists of a fixation system, a measurement and recording system, and an alignment system intended to measure the refractive power of the eye by measuring light reflexes from the retina.

Ophthalmic Rotary Prism   A Class I device with various prismatic powers intended to be hand-held and used to measure ocular deviation in patients with latent or manifest strabismus (eye muscle deviation).

Ophthalmic Sponge   A Class II device that is an absorbent sponge, pad, or spear made of folded gauze, cotton, cellulose, or other material intended to absorb fluids from the operative field in ophthalmic surgery.

Ophthalmic Surgical Marker   A Class I device intended to mark, by use of ink, dye, or indentation, the location of ocular or scleral surgical manipulation.

Ophthalmic Tantalum Clip   A malleable, metallic, Class II device intended to be implanted permanently or temporarily to bring together the edges of a wound to aid healing or prevent bleeding from small blood vessels in the eye.

Ophthalmic Trial Lens Clip   (1) A Class I device intended to reflect

Ophthalmic Trial Lens Frame

light for use in examination of the eye. (2) A Class I device intended to hold prisms, spheres, cylinders, or occluders on a trial frame or spectacles for vision testing.

Ophthalmic Trial Lens Frame   A mechanical Class I device intended to hold trial lenses for vision testing.

Ophthalmic Trial Lens Set   A Class II device that is a set of lenses of various dioptric powers intended to be hand-held or inserted in a trial frame for vision testing to determine refraction.

Ophthalmoscope   An AC-powered or battery-powered Class II device containing illumination and viewing optics intended to examine the media (cornea, aqueous, lens, and vitreous) and the retina of the eye.

Opiate Test System   A device intended to measure any of the addictive narcotic pain-relieving opiate drugs in blood, serum, urine, gastric contents, and saliva. An opiate is any natural or synthetic drug that has morphine-like pharmacological actions. The opiates include drugs such as morphine glucuronide, heroin, codeine, nalorphine, and meperidine. Measurements obtained by this device are used in the diagnosis and treatment of opiate use or overdose, and in monitoring the levels of opiate administration to ensure appropriate therapy.

Optical Vision Aid   A Class I device that consists of a magnifying lens, with an accompanying AC-powered or battery-powered light source, intended for use by a patient who has impaired vision to increase the apparent size of object detail.

Optokinetic Drum   A drum-like Class I device covered with alternating white and dark stripes or pictures that can be rotated on its handle. The device is intended to elicit and evaluate nystagmus (involuntary rapid movement of the eyeball) in patients.

Oral Cavity Evacuator   A Class I hand-held device that consists of a plastic tube attached to a suction unit and is used to remove fluids from the oral cavity during dental procedures.

Oral Irrigation Unit   A Class I AC-powered device intended to be used to remove food particles from between the teeth and promote good periodontal condition by means of a pressurized water stream.

Organ Bag   A Class I device that is a flexible plastic bag intended to be used as a temporary receptacle for an organ during surgical procedures to prevent moisture loss.

Ornithine Carbamyl Transferase Test System   A Class I device intended to measure the activity of the enzyme ornithine carbamyl transferase (OCT) in serum. Ornithine carbamyl transferase measurements are used in the diagnosis and treatment of liver diseases, such as infectious hepatitis, acute cholecystitis (inflammation of the gall bladder), cirrhosis, and liver metastases.

Orthodontic Band Driver A Class I spring-activated hand instrument that is used to place orthodontic bands on teeth. The device drives the band onto the tooth when the spring is released.

Orthodontic Band Material A Class I band material, such as stainless steel, that is used to construct a custom orthodontic band. The band is placed around a tooth that, because of its size and location, cannot be fitted with a preformed orthodontic band. The band provides a foundation for anchoring orthodontic appliances so that pressure can be exerted on the teeth.

Orthodontic Band Pusher A Class I bar-like stainless steel device used in orthodontic treatment to apply pressure on orthodontic bands in order to place the bands on teeth.

Orthodontic Band Setter A Class I bar-like device used in orthodontic treatment to position orthodontic bands on teeth.

Orthodontic Bracket Aligner A Class I plier-like device used to align brackets on orthodontic bands that are affixed to the teeth. To align the brackets, the gauge on the device is placed against the bottom edge of the tooth.

Orthodontic Elastic Band A Class I device made of rubber that is used with orthodontic appliances to alter the position of teeth by applying pressure on them.

Orthodontic Expansion Screw Retainer A Class I device used to exert pressure on the teeth during orthodontic treatment. The retainer has an adjustable screw that, when turned, expands the device laterally and, thereby, enlarges an area of the oral cavity, such as the palate.

Orthodontic Headgear (External) A Class I device that is used in conjunction with an orthodontic appliance to exert pressure on the teeth from outside the mouth. The headgear has a strap that wraps around the patient's neck or head and an inner bow portion that is fastened to the orthodontic appliance in the patient's mouth.

Orthodontic Ligature Tucking Instrument A Class I device used to push the end of a ligature under the arch wire so that soft tissues are not irritated by these ends. A ligature is the wire that fastens an orthodontic arch wire to the orthodontic band on a tooth.

Orthodontic Metal Bracket A Class I metal device that is welded to an orthodontic band or bonded to a tooth and that applies pressure from flexible orthodontic wire to the tooth in order to alter the position of the tooth.

Orthodontic Plastic Bracket A Class I plastic device that is bonded to a tooth and that applies pressure from a flexible orthodontic wire to the tooth in order to alter the position of the tooth.

Orthodontic Pliers   A Class I device used to shape and to adjust wires and bands in orthodontic treatment.

Orthodontic Preformed Band   A Class I prefabricated device made of metal. In orthodontic treatment, the device is affixed to a tooth to provide a foundation for anchoring orthodontic appliances so that pressure can be exerted on the teeth.

Orthodontic Space Maintainer (Preformed)   A Class I metal device that is used to preserve the space between teeth. The device is welded to the orthodontic bands affixed to the teeth adjacent to the space, which prevents movement of the adjacent teeth into the empty space.

Orthodontic Spring   A Class I metal device that is attached to the orthodontic bands affixed to the adjacent teeth and is used to apply pressure to teeth to correct their position.

Orthodontic Tube   A Class I metal device used in orthodontics to attach a wire or headgear to bands cemented to the teeth. The tube is welded to a band or bonded to the last tooth and allows insertion of an arch wire or headgear appliance.

Orthodontic Wire   A Class I device that is incorporated into an orthodontic appliance and is used to exert pressure on teeth in order to alter their position.

Orthodontic Wire Clamp   A Class I device that is attached to the arch wire to prevent movement of the arch wire.

Orthopedic Manual Surgical Instrument   A nonpowered, hand-held Class I device intended for medical purposes to manipulate tissue or for use with other devices in orthopedic surgery. This generic type of device includes the cerclage applier, awl, bender, drill brace, broach, bur, corkscrew, countersink, pin crimper, wire cutter, prosthesis driver, extractor, file, fork, needle holder, impactor, bending or contouring instrument, compression instrument, passer, socket positioner, probe, femoral neck punch, socket pusher, reamer, rongeur, scissors, screwdriver, bone skid, staple driver, bone screw starter, surgical stripper, tamp, bone tap, trephine, wire twister, and wrench.

Oscillometer   A Class II device used to measure physiological oscillations of any kind, e.g., changes in the volume of arteries.

Osmolality Test System   A Class I device intended to measure ionic and nonionic solute concentration in body fluids, such as serum and urine. Osmolality measurement is used as an adjunct to other tests in the evaluation of a variety of diseases, including kidney diseases (e.g., chronic progressive renal failure), diabetes insipidus, other endocrine and metabolic disorders, and fluid imbalances.

Osmometer for Clinical Use A Class I device intended to measure the osmotic pressure of body fluids. Osmotic pressure is the pressure required to prevent the passage of a solution with a lesser solute concentration into a solution with greater solute concentration when the two solutions are separated by a semipermeable membrane. The concentration of a solution affects its osmotic pressure, freezing point, and other physiochemical properties. Osmometers determine osmotic pressure by methods such as the measurement of the freezing point. Measurements obtained by this device are used in the diagnosis and treatment of body fluid disorders.

Osmotic Fragility Test A Class I device used to determine the resistance of red blood cells to hemolysis (destruction) in varying concentrations of hypotonic saline solutions.

Otoscope A Class I device intended to allow inspection of the external ear canal and tympanic membrane under magnification. The device provides illumination of the ear canal for observation by using an AC- or battery-powered light source and an optical magnifying system.

Ouchterlony Agar Plate for Clinical Use A Class I device containing an agar gel used to examine antigen-antibody reactions. In immunodiffusion, antibodies and antigens migrate toward each other through gel which originally contained neither of these reagents. As the reagents come in contact with each other, they combine to form a precipitate that is trapped in the gel matrix and is immobilized.

Over-the-Counter (OTC) Denture Cleanser A Class I device that consists of material in the form of a powder, tablet, or paste, that is used to remove debris from removable prosthetic dental appliances, such as bridges or dentures. The dental appliance is removed from the patient's mouth when the appliance is cleaned.

Over-the-Counter (OTC) Denture Cushion A Class III prefabricated or noncustom-made device consisting of material, such as wax or cotton fibers, that is intended to be applied to the entire base or inner surface of a denture before the denture is inserted in a patient's mouth. The device is used to improve temporarily the fit of a loose or uncomfortable denture and can be purchased over the counter.

Over-the-Counter (OTC) Denture Pad A Class III prefabricated or noncustom-made device consisting of material, such as wax or cotton fibers, that is intended to be applied to a portion of the base or inner surface of a denture before the denture is inserted in a patient's mouth. The device is used to temporarily soothe sore areas of the gums caused by an improperly fitting denture and can be purchased over the counter.

Over-the-Counter (OTC) Denture Reliner   A Class III device consisting of a material, such as plastic resin, that is intended to be applied as a permanent coating or lining on the base or tissue-contacting surface of a denture. The device is used to replace a worn denture lining and can be purchased over the counter.

Over-the-Counter (OTC) Denture Repair Kit   A Class III device consisting of material, such as a resin monomer system of powder and liquid glues, that is intended to be applied permanently to a denture to mend cracks or breaks. The device can be purchased over the counter.

Oxalate Test System   A Class I device intended to measure the concentration of oxalate in urine. Measurements of oxalate are used to aid in the diagnosis or treatment of urinary stones or certain other metabolic disorders.

Oximeter   A Class II device used to transmit radiation at a known wavelength through blood and to measure the blood-oxygen saturation based on the amount of reflected or scattered radiation. It may be used alone or in conjunction with a fiberoptic oximeter catheter.

Oxygen Gas Analyzer   A Class II diagnostic anesthesiology device used to measure the concentration of oxygen in a gas mixture. The device may use analytical techniques such as polarography, thermal conductivity, or mass spectrometry.

Oxygen Mask   A Class I device placed over the patient's nose and mouth to administer oxygen.

Oxygen Tent   A Class I nonpowered device that encloses the patient's head and upper body to contain delivered oxygen.

Oxygen Uptake Computer   A Class II diagnostic anesthesiology device used to compute the amount of oxygen consumed by the patient and may include components for determining expired gas volume and composition.

P

Pacemaker   A Class III electronic instrument for stimulating the heart in which the natural pacing mechanism has failed.

Pacemaker (External transcutaneous)   A Class III device used to supply a periodic electrical impulse intended to pace the heart. The device is usually applied to the surface of the chest through electrodes such as defibrillator paddles.

Pacemaker, External Pulse Generator   A Class III device that has a power supply and electronic circuits that produce electrical pulses to stimulate the heart. This device, which is used outside the body, is used as a temporary substitute for the heart's intrinsic pacing system until a permanent pacemaker can be implanted, or to control irregular heartbeats in patients following cardiac surgery or a myocardial infarction. The device may have adjustments for impulse strength, duration, R-wave sensitivity, and other pacing variables.

Pacemaker, Implantable Pulse Generator   A Class III device having a power supply and electronic circuits that produce a periodic electrical impulse to stimulate the heart. This device is used as a substitute for the heart's intrinsic pacing system to correct both intermittent and continuous cardiac rhythm disorders. This generic term includes triggered, inhibited, and asynchronous devices implanted in the human body.

Pacemaker, Indirect Gnerator Function Analyzer   A Class II electrically powered device used to determine pacemaker function or pacemaker battery function by periodically monitoring an implanted pacemaker's pulse rate and pulse width. The device is noninvasive, and it detects pacemaker pulse rate and width via external electrodes in contact with the patient's skin.

Pacemaker, Temporary   Any pacemaker intended for short-term use (usually a few days, and in most cases no longer than two weeks). Commonly used in heart-block patients awaiting permanent pacemaker implantation, or in patients recuperating from myocardial infarction.

Pacemaker, Transvenous   The most common type of pacemaker, whose implantation involves inserting the leads through a major vein (subclavian, cephalic, or external jugular). The pulse generator is implanted subcutaneously in the pectoral area and occasionally under the pectoralis major.

Pacemaker Charger   A Class II device used transcutaneously to charge the batteries of a rechargeable pacemaker.

Pacemaker Electrode Function Tester   A Class II device that is connected to an implanted pacemaker lead that supplies an accurately calibrated, variable pacing pulse for measuring the patient's pacing threshold and the intracardiac R-wave potential.

Pacemaker Electrodes, Permanent and Temporary   Class III devices that are flexible, insulated, electrical conductors with one end connected to a pacemaker pulse generator and the other end applied to the heart. The device is used to transmit a pacing electrical stimulus from the pulse generator to the heart and/or to transmit the electrical signal of the heart to the pulse generator.

Pacemaker Generator Function Analyzer A Class II device that is connected to a pacemaker pulse generator to test any or all of the generator's parameters, including pulse duration, pulse amplitude, pulse rate, and sensing threshold.

Pacemaker Lead Adaptor A Class III device used to adapt a pacemaker lead so that it can be connected to a pacemaker pulse generator produced by a different manufacturer.

Pacemaker Polymeric Mesh Bag (1) A Class II device used to hold a pacemaker pulse generator. By encouraging tissue ingrowth, it creates a stable implant environment for the generator. (2) A Class II device used to hold a pacemaker lead generator. It is designed to create a stable implant environment for the generator.

Pacemaker Programmer A Class III device used to change noninvasively one or more of the electrical operating characteristics of a pacemaker.

Pacemaker Pulse Generator (External programmable) A Class II device that can be programmed to produce one or more pulses at preselected intervals. This device is used in electrophysiological studies.

Pacemaker Repair and Replacement Materials Class III devices that are adhesives, sealants, screws, crimps, and other materials used to repair a pacemaker lead or to connect a pacemaker lead to a pacemaker lead generator.

Pacemaker Service Tools Class I devices, such as screwdrivers and Allen wrenches, used to repair a pacemaker lead or to reconnect a pacemaker generator.

Pacemaker Test Magnet A Class II device used to test an inhibited or triggered type of pacemaker pulse generator and cause an inhibited or triggered generator to revert to asynchronous operation.

Pantograph A Class I device that is attached to the head and is used to duplicate lower jaw movements to aid in the construction of restorative and prosthetic dental devices. A marking pen is attached to the lower jaw component of the device, and, as the mouth opens, the pen records on graph paper the angle between the upper and lower jaws.

Paper Saliva Absorber A Class I device made of paper that is used to absorb moisture from the oral cavity during dental procedures.

Paraffin Bath A Class II device composed of a metal tub to be filled with liquid paraffin (wax) maintained at an elevated temperature in which the appendages (e.g., hands or fingers) are placed to relieve pain and stiffness.

Parainfluenza Virus Serological Reagents Class I devices that consist of antigens and antisera used in serological tests to identify parainfluenza virus antibodies in a patient's serum. The identification aids in the diagnosis of parainfluenza virus infections and provides epidemiological information on diseases caused by these viruses. Parainfluenza viruses cause many respiratory illnesses ranging from the common cold to pneumonia.

Parathyroid Hormone Test System A Class II device intended to measure the levels of parathyroid hormone in serum and plasma. Measurements of parathyroid hormone levels are used in the differential diagnosis of hypercalcemia (abnormally high levels of calcium in the blood) and hypocalcemia (abnormally low levels of calcium in the blood) resulting from disorders of calcium metabolism.

Partial Osicular Replacement Prosthesis A Class II device intended to be implanted for the functional reconstruction of segments of the ossicular chain. This facilitates the conduction of sound waves from the tympanic membrane to the inner ear. The device is made of materials such as stainless steel, tantalum, polytetrafluoroethylene, polyethylene, polytetrafluoroethylene with carbon fiber composite, absorbable gelatin material, porous polyethylene, or from a combination of these materials.

Partial Thromboplastin Time Test A Class II device used for primary screening for coagulation abnormalities, for evaluation on the effect of therapy on procoagulant disorders, and as an assay for coagulation factor deficiencies of the intrinsic coagulation pathway.

Partially Fabricated Denture Kit A Class III device composed of connected, preformed teeth that is used in the construction of dentures. A denture base is constructed, using the patient's mouth as the mold, by partially polymerizing the resin denture base materials while the materials are in contact with the oral tissues. After the denture base is constructed, the connected, preformed teeth are inserted into the base.

Passive Tendon Prosthesis A Class II device intended to be implanted that is made of silicon elastomer or a polyester reinforced medical grade silicone elastomer and is intended for use in the surgical reconstruction of a flexor tendon of the hand. The device is implanted for a period of two to six months to aid growth of a new tendon sheath. The device is not intended as a permanent implant, or to function as a replacement for the ligament or tendon, or to function as a scaffold for soft tissue ingrowth.

Patch, Intracardiac and Pledget A Class II device made of polypropylene, Teflon®, or Dacron® fabric, placed in the heart and used to repair septal defects, to patch grafting, to repair tissue, and to buttress sutures.

Patient Care Reverse Isolation Chamber   A Class II device consisting of a room-like enclosure designed to prevent the entry of harmful airborne material. This device protects a patient who is undergoing treatment for burns or is lacking a normal immunosuppressive defense due to therapy or congenital abnormality. The device includes fans and air filters that maintain an atmosphere of clean air at a pressure greater than the air pressure outside the enclosure.

Patient Position Support   A Class II device used to maintain the position of an anesthetized patient during surgery.

Patient Scale   A Class I device used to measure the weight of a patient who cannot stand on a scale. This generic device includes devices placed under a bed or chair to weigh both the support and the patient, devices where the patient to be weighed is lifted by a sling from a bed, and devices where the patient to be weighed is placed on the scale platform. The device may operate mechanically or it may be AC-powered and may include transducers, electronic signal amplification, conditioning and display equipment.

Patient Transducer and Electrode Cable   A Class II device consisting of an electrical conductor used to transmit signals from, or power excitation to, patient-connected electrodes or transducers.

Peak-Flow Meter for Spirometry   A Class II diagnostic anesthesiology device used to measure a patient's maximum ventilatory flow rate.

Pediatric (Open) Hospital Bed   A Class II device consisting of a bed or crib, with fixed end rails and movable and latchable side rails, designed for the use of a pediatric patient. The contour or the bed surface may be adjustable.

Penile Inflatable Implant   A Class III device consisting of two inflatable cylinders implanted in the penis, connected to a reservoir containing radiopaque fluid implanted in the lower abdomen, and a subcutaneous manual pump implanted in the scrotum. The penis becomes rigid (erected) when the cylinders are voluntarily inflated, thus relieving erectile impotence.

Penile Rigidity Implant   A Class II device that consists of two inflatable cylinders implated in the penis, connected to a reservoir filled with radiopaque fluid implanted in the abdomen, and a subcutaneous manual pump implanted in the scrotum. When the cylinders are inflated, they provide rigidity to the penis. This device is used in the treatment of erectile impotence.

Percutaneous Catheter   A Class II device that is introduced into a vein or artery through the skin using a dilator and a sheath or guide wire.

Perimeter   An AC-powered or manual Class I device intended to determine the extent of the peripheral visual field of a patient. The device projects light on various points of a curved surface, and the patient indicates whether he or she sees the light.

Perinatal Monitoring System and Accessories A Class II device used to show graphically the relationship between maternal labor and the fetal heart rate by means of combining and coordinating uterine contraction and fetal heart monitors with appropriate displays. It is used to assist in the assessment of the well-being of mother and fetus during pregnancy, labor, and delivery. This generic type of device may include any of the devices subject to six other proposals. This generic type of device also includes the following accessories: central monitoring system and remote repeaters, signal and lysis and display equipment, patient and equipment supports and component parts.

Perineal Heater A Class II device designed to apply heat directly by contact, or indirectly from a radiant source, to the surface of the perineum (the area between the vulva and the anus) and is used to soothe or to help heal the perineum after an episiotomy (incision of the vulvar orifice for obstetrical purposes). Included in this generic type of device are those devices identified as "direct contact perineal heaters" and "noncontact radiant perineal heaters."

Perineometer A Class II device, an intravaginal, fluid-filled pouch, attached to an external manometer, used to measure the strength of perineal muscles by offering preselected resistance to a patient's voluntary contraction of these muscles. The device may be used in the diagnosis and therapy of urinary incontinence or sexual dysfuction through exercise.

Periodontic or Endodontic Irrigating Syringe A Class I device used for the irrigation of tissues in the mouth, such as gums, in periodontic therapy and root canals in teeth in endodontic therapy.

Peristaltic Pump A Class II pumping device using a rotating drum with rollers attached to the circumference that rotates with a cylinder. A flexible tube is positioned between the drum and the containing cylinder so that rotation of the drum causes the rollers to squeeze the tube, thus forcing a pumping action.

Peritoneal Dialysis A Class II device used as an artificial kidney for the treatment of renal failure or toxemic conditions. Consists of peritoneal access device, dialysis administration set, dialysate, and sometimes a water purification system. After installation in the peritoneal cavity, the fluid is allowed to remain so undesirable substances pass through the lining membranes into the dialysate. These substances are subsequently removed when the dialysate is drained from the peritoneal cavity.

Peritoneo-Venous Shunt A Class III implantable device consisting of a catheter and pressure-activated, one-way valve. The catheter is implanted with one end in the peritoneal cavity and the other in a large vein, thus enabling ascitic fluid in the peritoneal cavity to be drained into the venous system for the treatment of intractable ascites.

Permanent Magnet A nonelectric Class I device that generates a magnetic field intended to find and remove metallic foreign bodies from eye tissue.

Personnel Protective Shield A Class I device intended for medical purposes to protect the patient, the operator, or other persons from unnecessary exposure to radiation during radiologic procedures by providing an attenuating barrier to radiation. This generic type of device may include articles of clothing, furniture, and movable or stationary structures.

Permanent and Temporary Pacemaker Electrodes Class III devices that are flexible, insulated electrical conductors with one end connected to a pacemaker pulse generator and the other end applied to the heart. They are used to transmit a pacing electrical stimulus from the pulse generator to the heart and/or to transmit the electrical signal of the heart to the pulse generator.

pH Catheter Probe A Class II device that is a catheter fitted with a special tip for measuring blood pH.

Phacofragmentation System An AC-powered Class II device with a fragmenting needle intended for use in cataract surgery to disrupt a cataract with ultrasound and extract the cataract.

Phenobarbital Test System A Class II device intended to measure phenobarbital, an antiepileptic and sedative-hypnotic drug, in human specimens. Measurements obtained by this device are used in the diagnosis and treatment of phenobarbital use or overdose and in monitoring levels of phenobarbital to ensure appropriate therapy.

Phenothiazine Test System A Class II device intended to measure any of the drugs of the phenothiazine class in human specimens. Measurements obtained by this device are used in the diagnosis and treatment of phenothiazine use or overdose.

Phenylalanine Test System A Class II device intended to measure free phenylalanine (an amino acid) in serum, plasma, and urine. Measurements of phenylalanine are used in the diagnosis and treatment of congenital phenylketonuria, which, if untreated, may cause mental retardation.

Phonocardiograph A Class II device used to amplify or condition the signal received from a cardiac sound transducer. The device provides the excitation energy for the transducer, and provides a visual or audible display of cardiac sounds.

Phonocardiographic Monitor A Class II device designed to detect, measure, and graphically record fetal heart sound electronically and noninvasively, and to ascertain fetal conditions during labor. It includes signal analysis and display instrumentation, patient and equipment supports, and other ancillary components.

6-Phosphogluconate Dehydrogenase Test System   A Class I device intended to measure the activity of the enzyme 6-phosphogluconate dehydrogenase (6 PGD) in serum and erythrocytes. Measurements of 6-phosphogluconate dehydrogenase are used in the diagnosis and treatment of certain liver diseases, such as hepitis, and anemias.

Phosphohexose Isomerase Test System   A Class I device intended to measure the activity of the enzyme phosphohexose isomerase in serum. Measurements of phosphohexose isomerase are used in the diagnosis and treatment of muscle diseases, such as muscular dystrophy, liver diseases, such as hepatitis or cirrhosis, and metastatic carcinoma.

Phospholipid Test System   A Class I device intended to measure phospholipids in serum and plasma. Measurements of phospholipids are used in the diagnosis and treatment of disorders involving lipid (fat) metabolism.

Phosphorus (Inorganic) Test System   A Class I device intended to measure inorganic phosphorus in serum, plasma, and urine. Measurements of phosphorus (inorganic) are used in the diagnosis and treatment of various disorders, including parathyroid gland and kidney diseases, and vitamin D imbalance.

Photofluorographic X-ray System   A Class II device that includes a fluoroscopic X-ray unit and a camera intended to produce and photograph a fluoroscopic image of the body. This generic type of device may include signal analysis and display equipment, patient and equipment supports, component parts, and accessories.

Physical Therapy Muscle Relaxer   A motorized Class II device used to relieve minor muscle aches and pains. The generic type of device was considered under the name "powered massager."

Pipetting and Diluting System for Clinical Use   A Class I device intended to provide an accurately measured volume of liquid at a specified temperature for use in certain test procedures. This generic type of device system includes serial, manual, automated, and semiautomated dilutors, pipettors, dispensers, and pipetting stations.

Pit and Fissure Sealant and Conditioner   A Class II device composed of resin, such as polymethyl methacrylate, that is used primarily in young children to seal pit and fissure depressions in the biting surfaces of teeth in order to prevent cavities.

Plasma Oncometer for Clinical Use   A Class I device intended to measure plasma oncotic pressure, which is that portion of the total plasma osmotic pressure contributed by protein and other molecules too large to pass through a specified semipermeable membrane. Because variations in plasma oncotic pressure are indications of certain disorders, measurements of the variations are useful in the diagnosis and treatment of these disorders.

Plasma Oncometry Test System A Class I device intended to measure plasma oncotic pressure. Plasma oncotic pressure is that portion of the total fluid pressure contributed by proteins and other molecules too large to pass through a specified membrane. Measurements of plasma oncotic pressure are used in the diagnosis and treatment of dehydration and circulatory disorders related to low serum protein levels and increased capillary permeability, such as edema and shock.

Plasma Viscometer for Clinical Use A Class I device intended to measure the viscosity of plasma by determining the time period required for the plasma to flow a measured distance through a calibrated glass tube. Measurements obtained by this device are used to monitor changes in the amount of solids present in plasma in various disorders.

Plasminogen Immunological Test System A Class I device that consists of the reagents used to measure, by immunochemical techniques, the plasminogen (an inactive substance from which plasmin, a blood clotting factor, is formed) in serum, body fluids, and tissues. Measurement of plasminogen levels may aid in the diagnosis of fibrinolytic (blood-clotting) disorders.

Plastic Dental Filling Instrument A Class I device made of plastic that is used to carry filling material to the site of a restoration in the oral cavity.

Plastic Surgery Kit and Accessories A Class I device intended to be used to reconstruct maxillofacial deficiencies. The kit contains surgical instruments and materials used to make maxillofacial impressions before molding an external prosthesis.

Platelet Adhesion Test A Class I device used to determine in vitro platelet function.

Platelet Aggregometer A Class II device used to determine changes in platelet shape and platelet aggregation following the addition of an aggregating reagent to a platelet-rich plasma.

Plethysmograph, Impedance A Class II device used to estimate blood flow characteristics by measuring electrical impedance changes in a given region of the body.

Plethysmograph, Pressure A Class II device used to determine the airway resistance and lung volumes by measuring pressure changes while the patient is in an airtight box.

Plethysmograph, Volume A Class II device used to determine lung volume changes while the patient is maintained in an airtight chamber.

Plinth A Class I flat padded board with legs on which a patient is placed for treatment or examination.

PMAA (Premarket Approval Application) The medical device PMAA is the cousin of the New Drug Application (NDA) and results in a determination by the FDA that the device is safe and effective for its labelled indications. A PMAA is required for Class III devices, which include:

(1) Pre-1976 devices that were subsequently classified into Class III and devices that are substantially equivalent to these devices

(2) Pre-1976 devices that were regulated as new drugs

(3) Post-1976 devices that are not substantially equivalent to devices commercially available before the Medical Device Amendments were enacted

PMN (Premarket Notification), or 510(k) Provision The most used and one of the most critical provisions of the 1976 Medical Device Amendments. Under this process, a manufacturer is required to file with the FDA ninety days before a new device is to be marketed, a premarket notification demonstrating that the device is substantially equivalent to a device that was on the market prior to 1976 and is therefore marketable without formal FDA approval. In enacting Section 510(k), Congress divided medical devices into two broad categories: (1) Preamendment—those introduced into commercial distribution prior to May 28, 1976, and (2) Postamendment—those introduced into commercial distribution after May 28, 1976. Section 510(k) is used to notify the FDA in two situations: (1) When first marketing a device that is "substantially equivalent" to a preamendment device and (2) When changing a device in a way that could significantly affect safety or effectiveness. Examples of significant changes would be changes in design, material, composition, energy source, manufacturing process, or intended use. A premarket notification *is not an approval*. A letter from the FDA clearing a premarket notification is simply a determination by the FDA that the proposed device is substantially equivalent to a preamendment device and thus will be placed in the same class as the preamendment device. The FDA strictly prohibits any manufacturer from representing that a 510(k) is an "FDA approval."

Pneumatic Tourniquet Air-powered Class II device consisting of a pressure-regulating unit, connecting tubing, and an inflatable cuff. The cuff is intended to be wrapped around a patient's limb and inflated to reduce or totally occlude circulation during surgery.

Pneumoencephalographic Chair A Class II device consisting of a chair intended to support and position a patient during pneumo-encephalography (X-ray imaging of the brain).

Pneumotachometer A Class II device used to determine gas flow by measuring the pressure differential across a known resistance. The device may use a set of capillaries or a metal screen for the resistive element.

Poliovirus Serological Reagents Class I devices that consist of anti-gens and antisera used in serological tests to identify poliovirus antibodies in a patient's serum. Additionally, some of these reagents consist of poliovirus antisera conjugated with a fluorescent dye (immunofluorescent reagents) used to identify polioviruses from clinical specimens and/or from tissue culture isolates derived from clinical specimens. The identification aids in the diagnosis of poliomyelitis and provides epidemiological information on this disease. Poliomyelitis (polio) is an acute infectious disease that, in its serious form, affects the central nervous system. Poliovirus can destroy portions of the spinal cord motor neuron, causing debilitating paralysis.

Polishing Agent Strip A Class I device composed of a plastic strip to which an abrasive material is affixed. The device is used to polish restorative materials, such as amalgam or silicate, especially in areas between the teeth.

Polishing Wheel A Class I device composed of a material, such as hard rubber, that is used to polish restorative materials in readily accessible areas of the oral cavity. The device is held by a dental handpiece.

Polyacrylamide Polymer, Modified Cationic Denture Adhesive A Class III device composed of cationic polyacrylamide polymer that is applied to the base of a denture before the denture is inserted into the patient's mouth. The device is used to improve denture retention and comfort.

Polymethylmethacrylate (PMMA) Bone Cement (Luting agent) A Class III device intended to be implanted that is made from methylmethacrylate, polymethylmethacrylate, esters of methacrylic acid, or copolymers containing polymethylmethacrylate and polystyrene. The device is intended for use in arthroplastic procedures of the hip, knee, and other joints for the fixation of polymer or metallic prosthetic implants to the living bone.

Polymethylmethacrylate (PMMA) Diagnostic Contact Lens A Class II device that is a curved shell of PMMA intended to be applied for a short period of time directly on the globe or cornea of the eye for diagnosis or therapy of intraocular abnormalities.

Polytetrafluoroethylene with Carbon Fiber Composite Implant Material A porous Class II device material intended to be implanted during surgery of the chin, jaw, nose, or bones or tissue near the eye or ear. The device material serves as a space-occupying substance and is shaped and formed by the surgeon to conform to the patient's need.

Polytetrafluoroethylene (PTFE) Vitreous Carbon Material A Class II device composed of polytetrafluoroethylene and vitreous carbon that is used in maxillofacial alveolar ridge augmentation, and to coat metal surgical implants in the alveoli and the temporomandibular joints.

Polytetrafluoroethylene Injectable An injectable paste, prosthetic, Class III device composed of polytetrafluoroethylene intended to augment or reconstruct a vocal cord.

Polyvinylmethylether Maleic Acid Calcium-Sodium Double Salt Denture Adhesive A Class I device that is applied to the base of a denture before the denture is inserted into the patient's mouth. The device is used to improve denture retention and comfort.

Polyvinylmethylether Maleic Anhydride, Acid Calcium-Sodium Double Salt and Carboxymethylcellulose Sodium Denture Adhesive A Class I device that is applied to the base of a denture before the denture is inserted into the patient's mouth. The device is used to improve denture retention and comfort.

Polyvinylmethylether Maleic Anhydride, Acid Co-Polymer and Carboxymethylcellulose Sodium Denture Adhesive A Class I device that is applied to the base of a denture before the denture is inserted into the patient's mouth. The device is used to improve denture retention and comfort.

Porcelain Powder for Clinical Use A Class II device consisting of a mixture of kaolin, feldspar, quartz, or other substances that is used in the production of artificial teeth in fixed or removable denture, of jacket crowns, facings, and veneers. The device is used in restorative dentistry by heating the powder mixture to a high temperature in an oven to produce a hard prosthesis with a glass-like finish.

Porphobilinogen Test System A Class I device intended to measure porphobilinogen (one of the derivatives of hemoglobin that can make the urine a red color) in urine. Measurements obtained by this device are used in the diagnosis and treatment of porphyrias (primarily inherited diseases associated with disturbed porphyrine metabolism), lead poisoning, and other diseases characterized by alterations in the heme pathway.

Porphyrins Test System A Class I device intended to measure porphyrins (compounds formed during the biosynthesis of heme, a constituent of hemoglobin, and related compounds) in urine and feces. Measurements obtained by this device are used in the diagnosis and treatment of lead poisoning, porphyrias (primarily inherited diseases associated with disturbed porphyrin metabolism), and other diseases characterized by alterations in the heme pathway.

Portable Air Compressor A Class II device used to provide compressed air for medical use, e.g., to drive ventilators and other respiratory equipment.

Portable Leakage Current Alarm A Class II device used to measure the electrical leakage current between any two points of an electrical system, and to sound an alarm if the current exceeds a certain threshold.

Portable Liquid Oxygen Unit A Class II device that is a portable, thermally insulated container of liquid oxygen used for supplementation of a patient's inspired oxygen.

Portable Oxygen Generator A Class II device that uses either a chemical reaction or physical means (e.g., molecular sieve) to release oxygen for respiratory therapy.

Positive End Expiratory Pressure Breathing Attachment A Class II device attachment, connected to a ventilator, that is used to elevate pressure in a patient's lungs above atmospheric pressure at the end of exhalation.

Positron Camera A Class I device intended to image the distribution of positron-emitting radionuclides in the body. This generic type of device may include signal analysis and display equipment, patient and equipment supports, radionuclide anatomical markers, component parts, and accessories.

Posterior Artificial Teeth with Metal Insert A Class I device composed of porcelain that has a metal insert used to replace a natural tooth. The device is attached to surrounding teeth by a bridge and provides both an improvement in appearance and a functional occlusion that improves chewing ability.

Posture Chair for Cardiac and Pulmonary Treatment A Class I device used to assist in the rehabilitation and mobilization of patients with chronic heart and lung disease.

Potassium Test System A Class II device intended to measure potassium in serum, plasma, and urine. Measurements obtained by this device are used to monitor electrolyte balance in the diagnosis and treatment of disease conditions characterized by low or high blood potassium levels.

Potentiating Media for in vitro Diagnostic Use Class II devices that are media, such as bovine albumin, used to suspend red cells to enhance cell reactions for antigen-antibody testing.

Powered Algesimeter A Class II diagnostic anesthesiology device that uses electrical stimulation to determine a patient's sensitivity to pain following admininistration of anesthesia.

Powered Breast Pump An electrically powered, suction, Class II device used for pospartum extraction of milk from the breast.

Powered Communication System An electrical- or battery-powered Class II device used to transmit or receive information. It is used by persons unable to use their hands because of physical impairment. Examples of powered communication systems include the following: a specialized typewriter, a reading machine, and a video picture and word screen.

Powered Corneal Bur An AC-powered or battery-powered Class I device that is a motor and drilling tool intended to remove rust rings from the cornea of the eye.

Powered Environmental Control System An electrical- or battery-powered Class II device used by a patient to operate an environmental control function. Examples of environmental control functions include the following: to control room temperature, to answer a doorbell or telephone, or to sound an alarm for assistance.

Powered Exercise Equipment Motorized Class II devices used to redevelop muscles, restore motion to joints, and provide general physical conditioning. Examples of powered exercise equipment are the powered treadmill, the powered bicycle, and powered parallel bars.

Powered Flotation Therapy Bed A Class II device that may have an electrically heated mattress and is designed to accommodate a large volume of constantly moving water, air, mud, or sand in its mattress. This device is used as an aid to nursing care for the acceleration of healing or prevention of decubitus ulcers (bedsores), for patients with severe or extensive burns, or to aid circulation.

Powered Heating Pad An electrical Class II device used for dry-heat therapy of body surfaces. It is capable of maintaining an elevated temperature during use.

Powered Inflatable Tube Massager A powered Class II device used to relieve minor muscle aches and pains. It simulates kneading and stroking of tissues with the hands by use of an inflatable pressure cuff.

Powered Muscle Stimulator A motorized Class II device used to repeatedly contract muscles by passing electrical currents through electrodes contacting the affected body area.

Powered Myoelectric Biofeedback Equipment A Class II device that monitors certain bodily functions (e.g., muscle contraction relaxation, skin temperature, and electrical resistance of skin) and displays the output of the device to the patient. It is used to decrease psychophysiological symptoms and aid in muscle training performance. The device may be powered by alternating current (AC), or it may be battery powered.

Powered Nasal Irrigator An AC-powered Class I device intended to wash the nasal cavity by means of a pressure-controlled pulsating stream of water. The device consists of a control unit and pump connected to a spray tube and nozzle.

Powered Patient Rotation Bed A Class II device that turns a patient who is constrained to a reclining position. It is used to treat patients with severe or extensive burns, decubitus ulcers, urinary tract blockage, and to aid circulation.

Powered Patient Transport A Class II motorized device used to assist patient transfers to and from the bath, beds, chairs, treatment modalities, transport vehicles, and up and down flights of stairs.

Powered Radiation Therapy Patient Support Assembly An electrically powered Class II device composed of an adjustable couch intended to support a patient during radiation therapy.

Powered Reflex Hammer A motorized Class II device used to elicit and determine controlled deep tendon reflexes.

Powered Suction Pump A portable, AC-powered or compressed air-powered Class II device intended to remove infectious materials from wounds, or fluids from a patient's airway or respiratory support system. The device may be used during surgery in the operating room or at the patient's bedside. The device may include a microbial filter.

Powered Table A Class II device composed of an electrically operated flat surface table that can be adjusted to various positions. It is used by patients with circulatory neurological, or musculoskeletal conditions to increase tolerance to an upright or standing position.

Powered Toothbrush A Class I AC or battery-powered device intended to remove plaque or food particles from the teeth to reduce tooth decay. It consists of a handle containing a motor that provides vibrations to a toothbrush that is inserted in one end.

Powered Traction Equipment Class II devices used in conjunction with belts and harnesses to exert therapeutic tensile (pulling) forces on the body.

Powered Vaginal Muscle Stimulator An electrically powered device designed to stimulate directly the muscles of the vagina with pulsating electrical current. This device is used to increase muscular tone and strength in the treatment of sexual dysfunction. This generic type of device does not include devices used to treat urinary incontinence.

Powered Wheel Stretcher A Class II device composed of a battery-powered table with wheels that is used by patients who are unable to propel themselves independently, and who must maintain a prone or supine position for prolonged periods of time because of skin ulcers or contractures (muscle contractions).

Powered Wheelchair A battery-operated Class II device with wheels that is used to provide mobility to persons restricted to a sitting position.

Prealbumin Immunological Test System   A Class I device that consists of the reagents used to measure, by immunochemical techniques, the prealbumin (a plasma protein) in serum and other body fluids. Measurement of prealbumin levels in serum may aid in the assessment of the patient's nutritional status.

Precious Metal Alloy for Clinical Use   A Class II device that is a mixture of metals, the major components of which are silver and palladium. It may also contain smaller quantities of other metals, such as copper, gold, and platinum. It is used to fabricate dental appliances such as crowns and bridges.

Precision Attachment   A Class I device made of cast metal used in restorative dentistry in conjunction with removable partial dentures. Various forms of the device are used to connect a lower partial denture with another lower partial denture, to connect an upper partial denture with another upper partial denture, to connect either an upper or lower partial denture to a tooth or crown, or to connect a fixed bridge to a partial denture.

Predictive Pulmonary-Function Value Calculator   A Class II diagnostic anesthesiology device used to calculate pulmonary-function values based on empirical equations.

Preformed Anchor   A Class I prefabricated device made of metal, such as stainless steel or titanium, that is incorporated into a dental appliance, such as a denture, to help stabilize the appliance in the patient's mouth.

Preformed Bar   A Class I prefabricated device made of metal, such as heavy wire, wrought metal, or cast metal, that is incorporated into a dental appliance, such as denture, to connect the part to the dental appliance.

Preformed Clasp   A Class I prefabricated device made of cast metal, such as chrome-cobalt, that is incorporated into a dental appliance, such as a partial denture, to help stabilize the appliance in the patient's mouth by fastening the clamp to an adjacent tooth.

Preformed Crown   A Class I device made of plastic or metal that is affixed temporarily to a tooth after removal of, or breakage of, the natural crown. It is used as a functional restoration until a permanent crown is constructed. The device also is used as a functional restoration for a badly decayed, deciduous tooth until the adult tooth erupts.

Preformed Cusp   A Class I prefabricated device made of plastic that is used as a temporary cusp to achieve occlusal harmony prior to permanent restoration of the tooth.

Preformed Gold Denture Teeth A Class I device composed principally of gold metal and other metals that is used as a tooth or a portion of a tooth in a fixed or removable partial denture.

Preformed Impression Tray A Class I metal or plastic device used to hold impression material, such as alginate, during the making of an impression of a patient's teeth or alveolar process. The impression is used to reproduce the structure of a patient's teeth and gums.

Preformed Orthodontic Space Maintainer A Class I metal device that is used to preserve the space between the teeth. The device is welded to the orthodontic bands affixed to the teeth adjacent to the space, preventing movement of the adjacent teeth into the empty space.

Preformed Plastic Denture Teeth A Class II prefabricated device composed of materials, such as methyl methacrylate, that is used as a tooth in a denture.

Preformed Wire Clasp A Class II device made of bendable stainless steel wire that is incorporated into a dental appliance, such as an orthodontic retainer, and is used to anchor the appliance to a tooth.

Pregnanediol Test System A Class I device intended to measure pregnanediol (a major urinary metabolic product of progesterone) in urine. Measurements obtained by this device are used in the diagnosis and treatment of disorders of the ovaries or placenta.

Pregnanetriol Test System A Class I device intended to measure pregnanetriol (a precursor in the biosynthesis of the adrenal hormone cortisol) in urine. Measurements obtained by this device are used in the diagnosis and treatment of congenital adrenal hyperplasia (congenital enlargement of the adrenal gland).

Pregnenolone Test System A Class I device intended to measure pregnenolone (a precursor in the biosynthesis of the adrenal hormone cortisol and adrenal androgen) in serum and plasma. Measurements obtained by this device are used in the diagnosis and treatment of diseases of the adrenal cortex or the gonads.

Premarket Notification 510(k) See PMN.

Prescription Spectacle Lens A glass or plastic Class I device that is a lens intended to be worn by a patient in a spectacle frame to provide refractive corrections in accordance with a prescription for the patient. The device may be modified to protect the eyes from bright sunlight (i.e., prescription sunglasses). Prescription sunglass lenses may be reflective, tinted, polarizing, or photosensitized.

Pressure Infusor for I.V. Bag A Class II device consisting of an inflatable cuff that is placed around an I.V. bag. When the device is inflated, it increases the pressure on the I.V. bag to assist the infusion of the fluid.

Pressure Regulator   A Class II device often called a pressure reducing valve, that is used to convert a gas pressure from a high variable pressure to a lower, more constant working pressure. The device includes mechanical oxygen regulators.

Pressure Transducer   A Class II device used to measure the pressure between a device and soft tissue by converting pressure inputs to analog electrical signals.

Pressure Tubing and Accessories   Class II flexible or rigid devices used to deliver pressurized medical gases.

Pressure-Applying Device   A Class I device that is a table with an adjustable overhead weight attached. In place of the therapist's hands, a weight is placed on the back of a prone patient. It is used to apply continuous pressure to the paravertebral tissues with the intended purpose of providing muscular relaxation and neuro-inhibition.

Primidone Test System   A Class II device intended to measure primidone, an antiepileptic drug, on human specimens. Measurements obtained by this device are used in the diagnosis and treatment of primidone overdose and in monitoring levels of primidone to ensure appropriate therapy.

Processing System for Frozen Blood   A Class II device used to glycerolize red blood cells prior to freezing to minimize hemolysis (disruption of the red cell membrane accompanied by the release of hemoglobin) due to freezing and thawing of red blood cells, and to deglycerolize and wash thawed cells for subsequent reinfusion.

Progesterone Test System   A Class I device intended to measure progesterone (a female hormone) in serum and plasma. Measurements obtained by this device are used in the diagnosis and treatment of disorders of the ovaries or placenta.

Prolactin (Lactogen) Test System   A Class I device intended to measure the anterior pituitary polypeptide hormone prolactin in serum and plasma. Measurements obtained by this device are used in the diagnosis and treatment of disorders of the anterior pituitary gland or of the hypothalamus portion of the brain.

Properdin Factor B Immunological Test System   A Class II device that consists of the reagents used to measure, by immunochemical techniques, properdin factor B in serum and body fluids. The deposition of properdin factor B in body tissues, or a corresponding depression in the amount of properdin factor B in serum and body fluids, is evidence of the involvement of the alternative to the classical pathway of activation of complement (a group of plasma proteins which cause the destruction of cells which are foreign to the body). Measurement of properdin factor B aids in the diagnosis of several kidney diseases, e.g., chronic glomerulonephritis (inflammation of the glomeruli of the kidney), lupus nephritis (kidney disease asso-

159

ciated with a multisystem autoimmune disease, systemic lupus erythematosus), as well as several skin diseases, e.g., dermatitis herpetiformis (presence of vesicles on the skin that burn and itch) and pemphigus vulgaris (large vesicles on the skin). Other diseases in which the alternate pathway of complement activation has been implicated include rheumatoid arthritis, sickle cell anemia, and gram-negative bacteremia.

Prophylaxis Cup A Class I device made of rubber that is held by a dental handpiece and used to apply polishing agents during prophylaxis. The dental handpiece spins the rubber cup holding the polishing agent and the user applies it to the teeth to remove debris.

Propoxyphene Test System A Class II device intended to measure propoxyphene, a pain-relieving drug, in serum, plasma, and urine. Measurements obtained by this device are used in the diagnosis and treatment of propoxyphene use or overdose or in monitoring levels of propoxyphene to ensure appropriate therapy.

Prosthesis (Chin prosthesis) A Class II silicone rubber solid device intended to be implanted to augment or reconstruct the chin.

Prosthesis (Ear prosthesis) A Class II silicone rubber solid device intended to be implanted to reconstruct the external ear.

Prosthesis (Esophageal prosthesis) A plastic tube or tube-like Class III device that may have mesh reinforcement that is intended to be implanted in, or affixed externally to, the chest and throat to restore the esophagus or provide pharyngoesophageal continuity.

Prosthesis (Esophageal prosthesis [Taub design]) A Class II device intended to direct pulmonary air flow to the pharynx in the absence of the larynx, thereby permitting esophageal speech. The device is interposed between openings in the trachea and the esophagus and may be removed and replaced each day by the patient. During phonation, air from the lungs is directed to flow through the device and over the esophageal mucosa to provide a sound source that is articulated as speech.

Prosthesis (External aesthetic restoration prosthesis) A Class I device intended to be used to construct an external artificial body structure, such as an ear, breast, or nose. Usually the device is made of silicone rubber, and it may be fastened to the body with an external prosthesis adhesive. The device is not intended to be implanted.

Prosthesis (Mandibular implant facial prosthesis) A Class II device that is intended to be implanted for use in the functional reconstruction of mandibular deficits. The device is made of materials such as stainless steel, tantalum, titanium, cobalt-chromium based alloy, polytetrafluoroethylene, silicone elastomer, polyethylene, polyurethane, or polytetrafluoroethylene with carbon fiber composite.

Prosthesis (Nose prosthesis) A silicone rubber, solid, Class II device intended to be implanted to augment or reconstruct the nasal dorsum.

Prosthesis (Partial ossicular replacement prosthesis) A Class II device intended to be implanted for the functional reconstruction of segments of the ossicular chain and facilitates the conduction of sound waves from the tympanic membrane to the inner ear. The device is made of materials such as stainless steel, tantalum, polytetrafluoroethylene, polyethylene, polytetrafluoroethylene with carbon fiber composite, absorbable gelatin material, porous polyethylene, or from a combination of these materials.

Prosthesis (Silicon gel-filled breast prosthesis) Class III devices made of: (1) Single-lumen silicone gel-filled breast prosthesis. A single-lumen silicone gel-filled breast prosthesis is a silicone rubber shell made of polysiloxane(s), such as polydimethylsiloxane and polydiphenylsiloxane. The shell contains either a fixed amount cross-linked polymerized silicone gel, filler, and stabilizers, or is filled to the desired size with injectable silicone gel at time of implantation. The device is intended to be implanted to augment or reconstruct the female breast. (2) Double-lumen silicone gel-filled breast prosthesis. A double-lumen silicone gel-filled breast prosthesis is a silicone rubber inner shell and a silicone rubber outer shell. Both shells are made of polysiloxane(s), such as polydimethylsiloxane and polydiphenylsiloxane. The inner shell contains fixed amounts of cross-linked, polymerized silicone gel, fillers, and stabilizers. The outer shell is inflated to the desired size with sterile isotonic saline before or after implantation. The device is intended to be implanted to augment or reconstruct the female breast. (3) Polyurethane covered, silicone gel-filled breast prosthesis. A polyurethane covered, silicone gel-filled breast prosthesis is an inner silicone rubber shell made of polysiloxane(s), such as polydimethylsiloxane and polydiphenylsiloxane, with an outer silicone adhesive layer and an outer covering of polyurethane. Contained within the inner shell is a fixed amount of cross-linked polymerized silicone gel, fillers, and stabilizers, and an inert support structure compartmentalizing the silicone gel. The device is intended to be implanted to augment or reconstruct the female breast. Note: Date premarket approval application (PMA) is required. PMA's are required to be filed with the Food and Drug Administration from July 9, 1991 for any silicone gel-filled breast prothesis that was in commercial distribution before May 28, 1976, or that has on or before July 9, 1991, been found to be substantially equivalent to a silicone gel-filled breast prosthesis that was in commercial distribution before May 28, 1976. Any other silicone gel-filled breast prosthesis shall have an approved PMA in effect before being placed in commercial distribution.

Prosthesis (Silicone inflatable breast prosthesis) A Class III device composed of a silicone rubber shell made of polysiloxane(s), such as polydimethylsiloxane and polydiphenylsiloxane, that is inflated to the desired size with sterile isotonic saline before or after implantation. The device is intended to be implanted to augment or reconstruct the female breast.

Prosthesis (Total ossicular replacement prosthesis) A Class II device intended to be implanted for the total functional reconstruction of the ossicular chain, and facilitates the conduction of sound waves from the tympanic membrane to the inner ear. The device is made of materials such as polytetrafluoroethylene, polytetrafluoroethylene with vitreous carbon fiber composite, porous polyethylene, or from a combination of these materials.

Prosthesis (Tracheal prosthesis) A tubular Class III device intended to be implanted to reconstruct the trachea.

Prosthesis Modification Instrument for Ossicular Replacement Surgery A Class I device intended for use by a surgeon to construct ossicular replacements. This generic type of device includes the ear, nose, and throat cutting block, wire crimper, wire bending die; wire closure forceps; piston cutting jib gelfoam TM punch; wire cutting scissors; and ossicular finger vise.

Prosthetic Heart Valve Holder A Class II device used to hold a replacement heart valve while it is being sutured into place.

Prosthetic Heart Valve Sizer A Class II device used to measure the size of the natural valve opening to determine the size of the appropriate replacement heart valve.

Protein (Fractionation) Test System: A Class I device intended to measure protein fractions in blood, urine, cerebrospinal fluid, and other body fluids. Protein fractionations are used as an aid in recognizing abnormal proteins in body fluids and genetic variants of proteins produced in diseases with tissue destruction.

Prosthetic and Orthotic Accessories A Class I device used to support, protect, or aid in the use of a cast, orthosis (brace), or prosthesis. Examples of prosthetic and orthotic accessories include the following: a pelvic support band and belt, a cast shoe, a limb cover, a prosthesis alignment device, a postsurgical pylon, a transverse rotator, or a temporary training splint.

Protein-Bound Iodine Test System A Class I device intended to measure protein-bound iodine in serum. Measurements of protein-bound iodine obtained by this device are used in the diagnosis and treatment of thyroid disorders.

Proteus spp. (Weil-Felix) Serological Reagents Class I devices that consist of antigens and antisera, including antisera conjugated with a fluorescent dye (immunofluorescent reagents), derived from the bacterium *Proteus vulgaris* used in agglutination tests (a specific type of antigen-antibody reaction) for the detection of antibodies to rickettsia (virus-like bacteria) in a patient's serum. Test results aid in the diagnosis of diseases caused by rickettsia, such as typhus fever and rocky mountain spotted fever, and provide epidemiologic information on these diseases.

Prothrombin Consumption Test A Class II device that measures the patient's capacity to generate thromboplastin in the coagulation process. The test also is an indirect indicator of qualitative or quantitative platelet abnormalities. It is a screening test for thrombocytopenia (decreased number of blood platelets) and hemophilia A and B.

Prothrombin Immunological Test System A Class I device that consists of the reagents used to measure, by immunochemical techniques, the prothrombin (clotting factor II) in serum. Measurements of the amount of antigenically competent (ability to react with protein antibodies) prothrombin aid in the diagnosis of patients with blood-clotting disorders.

Prothrombin Time Test A Class II device used as a general screening procedure for the detection of possible clotting factor deficiencies in the extrinsic coagulation pathway, which involves the reaction between coagulation factors III and VII, and to monitor patients receiving coumarin therapy (the administration of one of the coumarin anticoagulants in the treatment of venous thrombosis or pulmonary embolism.

Prothrombin-Proconvertin Test and Thrombotest Class II devices used in the regulation of coumarin therapy (administration of a coumarin anticoagulant such as sodium warfarin in the treatment of venous thrombosis and pulmonary embolism) and as a diagnostic test in conjunction with, or in place of, the quick prothrombin time test to detect coagulation disorders.

Protractor for Clinical Use A Class I device intended for use in measuring the angles of bones, such as on X-rays or in surgery.

***Pseudomonas* spp. Serological Reagents** Class II devices that consist of antigens and antisera, including antisera conjugated with a fluorescent dye (immunofluorescent reagents) used to identify *Pseudomonas* spp. from clinical specimens and/or from culture isolates derived from clinical specimens. The identification aids in the diagnosis of disease caused by bacteria belonging to the genus *Pseudomonas*. *Pseudomonas aeruginosa* is a major cause of hospital-acquired infections, and has been associated with urinary tract infections, eye infections, burn and wound infections, blood poisoning, abscesses, meningitis (inflammation of brain membranes), and melioidosis (a chronic pneumonia).

163

Ptosis Crutch   A Class I device intended to be mounted on the spectacles of a patient who has ptosis (drooping of the upper eyelid as a result of faulty development or paralysis) to hold the upper eyelid open.

Pulmonary-Function Data Calculator   A Class II diagnostic anesthesiology device used to calculate pulmonary-function values based on actual physical data obtained during pulmonary-function testing.

Pulp Tester   An AC- or battery-powered Class II device, used to evaluate the pulpal vitality of teeth by employing high frequency current, transmitted by an electrode, to stimulate the nerve tissue in the dental pulp.

Pump (Powered suction pump)   A portable, AC-powered or compressed air–powered Class II device intended to be used to remove infectious materials from wounds, or fluids from a patient's airway or respiratory support system. The device may be used during surgery in the operating room or at the patient's bedside. The device may include a microbial filter.

Pump (Withdrawal-infusion)   A Class II device designed to accurately inject medications into the bloodstream and to withdraw blood samples for use in determining cardiac output.

Pupillograph   An AC-powered Class I device intended to measure the pupil of the eye by reflected light and to record the responses of the pupil.

Pupillometer   An AC-powered or manual Class I device intended to measure, by reflected light, the width or diameter of the pupil of the eye.

Pyruvate Kinase Test System   A Class I device intended to measure the activity of the enzyme pyruvate kinase in erythrocytes (red blood cells). Measurements obtained by this device are used in the diagnosis and treatment of various inherited anemias due to pyruvate kinase deficiency or of acute leukemias.

Pyruvic Acid Test System   A Class I device intended to measure pyruvic acid (an intermediate compound in the metabolism of carbohydrate) in plasma. Measurements obtained by this device are used in the evaluation of electrolyte metabolism and in the diagnosis and treatment of acid-base and electrolyte disturbances or anoxia (the reduction of oxygen in body tissues).

Q

Qualitative and Quantitative Factor Deficiency Test   A Class II device used to diagnose specific coagulation defects, to monitor certain types of therapy, to detect coagulation inhibitors, and to detect a carrier state (a person carrying both a recessive gene for a coagulation factor deficiency, such as hemophilia, and the corresponding normal gene).

Quality Control Kit for Blood Banking Reagents   A Class II device that consists of sera, cells, buffers, and antibodies used to determine the specificity, potency, and reactivity of the cells and reagents used for blood banking.

Quality Control Kit for Culture Media   A Class I device that consists of paper disks, each impregnated with a specified, freeze-dried viable microorganism, used to determine if a given culture medium is able to support the growth of that microorganism(s). The device aids in the diagnosis of disease caused by pathogenic microorganisms and also provides epidemiological information on these diseases.

Quality Control Material (Assayed and unassayed) for Clinical Chemistry   A Class I device intended for medical purposes for use in a test system to estimate test precision and to detect systematic analytical deviations that may arise from reagent or analytical instrument variation. A quality control material (assayed or unassayed) may be used for proficiency testing in interlaboratory surveys. This generic type of device includes controls (assayed and unassayed) for blood gases, electrolytes, enzymes, multianalytes (all kinds), single (specified) analytes, or urinalysis controls.

Quinine Test System   A Class I device intended to measure quinine, a fever-reducing and pain-relieving drug intended for the treatment of malaria, in serum and urine. Measurements obtained by this device are used in the diagnosis and treatment of quinine overdose and malaria.

R

Rabiesvirus Immunofluorescent Reagents   Class II devices that consist of rabiesvirus antisera conjugated with a fluorescent dye used to identify rabiesviruses in specimens taken from suspected rabid animals. The identification aids in the diagnosis of rabies in patients exposed by animal bite and provides epidemiological information on rabies. Rabies is an acute infectious disease of the central nervous system that, if undiagnosed, may be fatal. The disease is commonly transmitted to humans by a bite from a rabid animal.

Radial Immunodiffusion Plate for Clinical Use   A Class I device that consists of a plastic plate to which agar gel containing antisera is added. In radial immunodiffusion, antigens migrate through gel that originally contains specific antibodies. As the reagents come in contact with each other they combine to form a precipitate that is trapped in the gel matrix and immobilized.

Radiation Therapy Beam-Shaping Block   A Class II device made of a highly attenuating material (such as lead) intended for medical purposes to modify the shape of a beam from a radiation therapy source.

Radiation Therapy Simulation System   A Class II fluoroscopic or radiographic X-ray system intended for use in localizing the volume to be exposed during radiation therapy and confirming the position and size of the therapeutic irradiation field produced. This generic type of device may include signal analysis and display equipment, patient and equipment supports, treatment planning computer programs, component parts, and accessories.

Radioallergosorbent (RAST) Immunological Test System   A Class II device that consists of the reagents used to measure, by immunochemical techniques, the allergen antibodies (antibodies which cause an allergic reaction) specific for a given allergen. Measurement of specific allergen antibodies may aid in the diagnosis of asthma, allergies, and other pulmonary disorders.

Radiofrequency Electrosurgical Cautery Apparatus   An AC-powered or battery-powered Class II device intended for use during ocular surgery to coagulate tissue or arrest bleeding by a high frequency electric current.

Radiofrequency Physiological Signal (Transmitters and receivers)   A Class II device used to condition a physiological signal so that it can be transmitted via radiofrequency from one location to another, e.g., a central monitoring station. The received signal is conditioned by the device into its original format so that it can be displayed.

Radiographic Anthropomorphic Phantom   A Class I device intended for medical purposes to simulate a human body for positioning radiographic equipment.

Radiographic ECG/Respirator Synchronizer   A Class I device intended to be used to coordinate an X-ray film exposure with the signal from an electrocardiograph (ECG) or respirator at a predetermined phase of the cardiac or respiratory cycle.

Radiographic Film   A Class I device that consists of a thin sheet of radiotransparent material, coated on one or both sides with a photographic emulsion, intended to record images during diagnostic radiologic procedures.

Radiographic Film Cassette   A Class II device intended for use during diagnostic X-ray procedures to hold a radiographic film in close contact with an X-ray intensifying screen and to provide a light-proof enclosure for direct exposure of radiographic film.

Radiographic Film/Cassette Changer   A Class II device intended to be used during a radiologic procedure to move a radiographic film or cassette between X-ray exposures and to position it during the exposure.

Radiographic Film/Cassette Changer Programmer   A Class II device intended to be used to control the operations of a film or cassette changer during serial medical radiography.

Radiographic Film Illuminator   A Class I device containing a visible light source covered with a translucent front that is intended to be used to view medical radiographs.

Radiographic Film Marking System   A Class I device intended for medical purposes to add identification and other information onto radiographic film by means of exposure to visible light.

Radiographic Grid   A Class I device that consists of alternating radiolucent and radiopaque strips intended to be placed between the patient and the image receptor to reduce the amount of scattered radiation reaching the image receptor.

Radiographic Head Holder   A Class I device intended to position the patient's head during a radiographic procedure.

Radiographic Intensifying Screen   A Class I device that is a thin, radiolucent sheet coated with a luminescent material that transforms incident X-ray photons into visible light and is intended, for medical purposes, to expose radiographic film.

Radiologic Patient Cradle   A Class II support device intended to be used for rotational positioning about the longitudinal axis of a patient during radiologic procedures.

Radiologic Quality Assurance Instrument   A Class I device intended, for medical purposes, to measure a physical characteristic associated with another radiologic device.

Radiologic Table   A Class II device intended, for medical purposes, to support a patient during radiologic procedures. The table may be fixed or tilting and may be electrically powered.

Radionuclide Radiation Therapy System   A Class II device intended to permit an operator to administer gamma radiation therapy with the radiation source located at a distance from the patient's body. This generic type of device may include signal analysis and display equipment, patient and equipment supports, treatment planning computer programs, component parts (including beam-limiting devices), and accessories.

Radionuclide Brachytherapy Source   A Class II device that consists of a radionuclide which may be enclosed in a sealed container made of gold, titanium, stainless steel, or platinum, and intended, for medical purposes, to be placed onto a body surface or into a body cavity or tissue as a source of nuclear radiation for therapy.

Radionuclide Dose Calibrator   A radiation detection Class II device intended to assay radionuclides before their administration to patients.

Radionuclide Rebreathing System   A Class II device intended to contain a gaseous or volatile radionuclide or a radionuclide-labelled aerosol, and permit it to be respired by the patient during nuclear medicine ventilatory tests (testing process of exchange between the lungs and the atmosphere). This generic type of device may include signal analysis and display equipment, patient and equipment supports, component parts, and accessories.

Radionuclide Teletherapy Source   A Class I device consisting of a radionuclide enclosed in a sealed container. The device is intended for radiation therapy with the radiation source located at a distance from the patient's body.

Radionuclide Test Pattern Phantom   A Class I device that consists of an arrangement of radiopaque or radioactive material sealed in a solid pattern that is intended to serve as a test for a performance characteristic of a nuclear medicine imaging device.

Rebreathing Device   A Class II device that enables the patient to rebreathe exhaled gases. It may be used in conjunction with pulmonary function testing or for increasing minute ventilation.

Recirculating Air Cleaner   A Class II device used to remove particles from the air by electrostatic precipitation or filtration.

Recorder (Medical magnetic tape)   A Class II device used to record and play back signals from, for example, physiological amplifiers, signal conditioners, or computers.

Recorder, Paper Chart   A Class II device used to print on paper and create a permanent record of, for example, a physiological signal amplifier, signal conditioner, or computer.

Rectal Dilator   A Class II device designed to dilate the anal sphincter and canal when the size of the anal opening may interfere with its function or the passage of an examining instrument.

Red Cell Indices Device   A red cell indices Class II device, usually part of a larger system, calculates or directly measures the erythrocyte mean corpuscular volume (MCV), the mean corpuscular hemoglobin (MCH), and the mean corpuscular hemoglobin concentration (MCHC). The red cell indices are used for the differential diagnosis of anemias.

Red Cell Lysing Reagent   A Class I device used to lyse (destroy) red blood cells for hemoglobin determinations or to remove red blood cells to facilitate the counting of white blood cells.

Red Cell Survival Test A device system used to measure the mean red cell survival or loss in either a patient or a suitable recipient.

Refractometer for Clinical Use A Class I device intended to determine the amount of solute in a solution by measuring the index of refraction (the ratio of the velocity of light in a vacuum to the velocity of light in the solution). The index of refraction is used to measure the concentration of certain analytes (solutes), such as plasma total proteins and urinary total solids. Measurements obtained by this device are used in the diagnosis and treatment of certain conditions.

Remote Controlled Radionuclide Applicator System An electromechanical or pneumatic Class II device intended to enable an operator to apply, by remote control, a radionuclide source into the body or to the surface of the body for radiation therapy. This generic type of device may include patient and equipment supports, component parts, treatment planning computer programs, and accessories.

Removable Skin Clip A clip-like Class I device intended to connect skin tissues temporarily to aid healing. It is not absorbable.

Removable Skin Staple A staple-like Class I device intended to connect external tissues temporarily to aid healing. It is not absorbable.

Reovirus Serological Reagents Class I devices that consist of antigens and antisera used in serological tests to identify reovirus antibodies in a patient's serum. The identification aids in the diagnosis of reovirus infections and provides epidemiological information on diseases caused by these viruses. Reoviruses are thought to cause only mild respiratory and gastrointestinal illnesses.

Replacement Heart Valve A Class III device intended to perform the function of any of the heart's natural valves. This generic device class includes valves constructed of prosthetic materials, biologic valves (e.g., porcine xenograft valves), or valves constructed of a combination of prosthetic and biologic materials.

Reservoir Bag A Class II device, usually made of conductive rubber, used in a breathing circuit as a reservoir for breathing gas and to assist, control, and monitor a patient's ventilation.

Resin Applicator A Class I brush-like device that is used to spread dental resin on a tooth prior to application of tooth shade material.

Resin Impression Tray Material A Class I device used in a two-step dental mold fabricating process. The device consists of a resin material, such as methyl methacrylate, and is used to form a cushion impression tray for use in cases in which a preformed impression tray is not suitable, such as in the fabrication of crowns, bridges, or full dentures. A preliminary impression in tray material is applied to this preliminary study model to form a custom tray.

This tray is then filled with impression material and inserted into the patient's mouth to make an impression from which a final, more precise model of the patient's mouth is cast.

Resin Tooth Bonding Agent   A Class I device, such as methylmethacrylate, that is painted on the interior of a prepared cavity of a tooth to improve retention of a restoration, such as a filling.

Respiratory Gas Humidifier   A Class II device used to add moisture, and sometimes, warm, breathing gases to the patient. Cascade, gas, heated, and prefilled humidifiers are included in this generic type of device.

Respiratory Syncytial Virus Serological Reagents   Class I devices that consist of antigens and antisera used in serological tests to identify respiratory syncytial virus antibodies in a patient's serum. Additionally, some of these reagents consist of respiratory syncytial virus antisera conjugated with a fluorescent dye (immunofluorescent reagents) and used to identify respiratory syncytial viruses from clinical specimens and/or from tissue culture isolates derived from clinical specimens. The identification aids in the diagnosis of respiratory syncytial virus infections and provides epidemiological information on diseases caused by these viruses. Respiratory syncytial viruses cause a number of respiratory tract infections, including the common cold, pharyngitis, and infantile bronchopneumonia.

Restorative or Impression Material Syringe   A Class I device used in the placement of impression material (alginate) or restorative material (amalgam) in the oral cavity. It consists of a hollow tube syringe body with a plunger at one end and a narrow opening at the opposite end through which the impression or restorative material is forced by the plunger.

Retentive and Splinting Pin   A Class I device made of a material, such as titanium, that is placed permanently in a tooth to provide retention and stabilization for a restoration, such as a crown, or to join two or more teeth together.

Retinol-Binding Protein Immunological Test System   A Class I device that consists of the reagents used to measure, by immunochemical techniques, retinol-binding protein that binds and transports vitamin A in serum and urine. Measurements of this protein may aid in the diagnosis of kidney disease and in monitoring patients with kidney transplants.

Retinoscope   An AC-powered or battery-powered Class I device intended to measure the refraction of the eye by illuminating the retina and noting the direction of movement of the light on the retinal surface and of the refraction by the eye of the emergent rays.

Retractor (Gastroenterology-urology fiberoptic)   A Class I device that consists of a mechanical retractor with a fiberoptic light system that is used to illuminate deep surgical sites.

Rheumatoid Factor Immunological Test System   A Class II device that consists of the reagents used to measure, by immunochemical techniques, the rheumatoid factor (antibodies to immunoglobulins) in human serum, body fluids, and tissues. Measurement of rheumatoid factor may aid in the diagnosis of rheumatoid arthritis.

Rhinovirus Serological Reagents   Class I devices that consist of the antigens and antisera used in serological tests to identify rhinovirus antibodies in a patient's serum. The identification aids in the diagnosis of rhinovirus infections and provides epidemiological information on diseases caused by these viruses. Rhinoviruses cause common colds.

Ribdam   A Class II device consisting of a broad strip of latex with supporting ribs used to drain surgical wounds where copious urine drainage is expected.

Rickettsia Serological Reagents   Class I device that consist of antigens and antisera used in serological tests to identify rickettsial antibodies in a patient's serum. Additionally, some of these reagents consist of rickettsial antisera conjugated with a fluorescent dye (immunofluorescent reagents) used to identify rickettsia directly from clinical specimens as well as to detect rickettsial antibodies in a patient's serum. The identification aids in the diagnosis of diseases caused by bacteria belonging to the genus *Rickettsiae* and provides epidemiological information on rickettsial diseases. Rickettsia are generally transmitted by arthropods (e.g., ticks and mosquitoes) and produce infections in humans characterized by rash and fever (e.g., typhus fever, spotted fever, Q fever, and trench fever).

Rigid Gas Permeable Contact Lens   A Class III device intended to be worn directly against the cornea of the eye to correct vision conditions. The device is made of various materials, such as cellulose acetate butyrate, acrylate-silicone, or silicone elastomers, whose main polymer molecules generally do not absorb or attract water.

Rigid Gas Permeable Contact Lens Solution   A Class III device intended to clean, disinfect, wet, or store a rigid gas permeable contact lens.

Rigid Pneumatic Structure Orthosis   A Class III device used to provide whole body support by means of a pressurized suit to help thoracic paraplegics walk.

Rocket Immunoelectrophoresis Equipment for Clinical Use   A Class I device used to perform a specific test on proteins by using a procedure called rocket immunoeletrophoresis. In this procedure an electric current causes the protein in a solution to migrate through agar gel containing specific antisera. The protein precipitates with the antisera in a rocket-shaped pattern giving the name to the device. The height of the peak (or the area under the peak) is proportional to the concentration of the protein.

Rocking Bed   A Class II device used to temporarily help patient ventilation by repeatedly tilting the patient, thereby using the weight of the abdominal contents to move the diphragm.

Roller-Type Cardiopulmonary Bypass Blood Pump   A Class II device that uses a roller mechanism to pump the blood through the cardiopulmonary bypass circuit during bypass surgery.

Root Canal Filling Resin   A Class I device composed of a material, such as methyl methacrylate, that is used during endodontic therapy to fill the root canal of a tooth.

Root Canal Post   A Class I metal device that is connected into the root canal of a tooth to stabilize and support a restoration.

Rubber Dam   A Class I device composed of a thin sheet of latex with a hole in the center that is used to isolate a tooth from fluids in the mouth during dental procedures, such as filling a cavity. The device is stretched around a tooth by inserting the tooth through the hole in the center.

Rubber Dam Clamp   A Class I device used to anchor a rubber dam (a barrier used to isolate a tooth from the fluids in the mouth during dental procedures, such as filling a cavity).

Rubber Dam Frame   A Class I device used to stretch and apply a rubber dam (a barrier used to isolate a tooth from the fluids in the mouth during dental procedures, such as filling a cavity).

Rubber Tip for Oral Hygiene   A Class I device made of rubber intended to stimulate and massage the gums to promote good periodontal condition. It is attached to a metal or plastic handle or to the handle of a toothbrush.

Rubella Virus Serological Reagents   Class II devices that consist of antigens and antisera used in serological tests to identify rubella virus antibodies in a patient's serum. The identification aids in the diagnosis of rubella (German measles) or confirmation of a person's immune status from past infections or immunizations and provides epidemiological information on German measles. Newborns who have been infected with rubella virus in the uterus may be born with multiple congenital defects (rubella syndrome).

Rubeola (Measles) Virus Serological Reagents   Class I devices that consist of antigens and antisera used in serological tests to identify rubeola (measles) virus antibodies in a patient's serum. The identification aids in the diagnosis of measles and provides epidemiological information on measles. Measles is an acute, highly infectious disease, particularly in children, characterized by a confluent and blotchy rash.

Russell Viper Venom Reagent   A Class I device used to determine the cause of an increase in the prothrombin time.

S

Sacculotomy Tack (Cody tack)   A Class II device that consists of a pointed stainless steel tack intended to be implanted to relieve the symptoms of vertigo. The device repetitively ruptures the utricular membrane as the membrane expands under increased endolymphatic pressure.

Salicylate Test System   A device intended to measure salicylates in human specimens. Salicylates are a class of analgesic, antipyretic, and anti-inflammatory drugs that includes aspirin. Measurements obtained by this device are used in diagnosis and treatment of salicylate overdose and in monitoring salicylate levels to ensure appropriate therapy.

Saliva Ejector Mouthpiece   A Class I device consisting of a plastic tube that is used to remove saliva continuously from the oral cavity during dental treatment. The tube is looped over the lips and is attached to a suction unit.

***Salmonella* spp. Serological Reagents**   Class II devices that consist of antigens and antisera used in serological tests to identify *Salmonella* spp. from cultured isolates derived from clinical specimens. Additionally, some of these reagents consist of antisera conjugated with a fluorescent dye (immunofluorescent reagents) used to directly identify *Salmonella* spp. from clinical specimens and/or cultured isolates derived from clinical specimens. The identification aids in the diagnosis of salmonellosis caused by bacteria belonging to the genus *Salmonella* and provides epidemiological information on this disease. Salmonellosis is characterized by high grade fever (enteric fever), severe diarrhea, and cramps.

Scale (Patient)   A Class I device used to measure the weight of a patient who cannot stand on a scale. This generic device includes devices placed under a bed or chair to weigh both the support and the patient, devices where the patient to be weighed is lifted by a sling from a bed, and devices where the patient to be weighed is placed on a scale platform. The device may operate mechanically or it may be AC-powered and may include transducers, electronic signal amplification, conditioning, and display equipment.

Scale (Stand-on patient)   A Class I device used to weigh a patient who is able to stand on the scale platform.

Scale (Surgical sponge) A nonelectrically powered Class I device used to weigh surgical sponges that have been used to absorb blood during surgery so that, by comparison with the known dry weight of the sponges, an estimate may be made of the blood lost by a patient during surgery.

Scaler (Rotary) A Class II abrasive device that is attached to a powered handpiece and is used to remove calculus deposits from teeth during dental cleaning and periodontal (gum) therapy.

Scaler (Ultrasonic) A Class II device used during dental cleaning and periodontal (gum) therapy to remove calculus deposits from teeth by application of an ultrasonically vibrating scaler tip to the teeth.

Scavenging Mask A Class II device positioned over the patient's nose to deliver anesthetic or analgesic gases to the upper airway and to remove excess and exhaled gas. It is used during dental procedures.

Scented, Deodorized, Menstrual Pad A Class II device made of an absorbent cotton or synthetic material pad with fragrant chemicals added for the purpose of deodorizing or for anesthetic purposes. The device is used to absorb menstrual or other vaginal discharge. This generic type of device does not include devices with added drugs or antimicrobial agents.

Scented, Deodorized, Menstrual Tampon A Class II device made of an absorbent cotton or synthetic material plug, inserted into the vagina, that is used to absorb menstrual or other vaginal discharge. It has fragrant chemicals added for the purpose of deodorizing or for aesthetic purposes. This generic type of device does not include devices with added drug or antimicrobial agents.

Schirmer Strip A Class I device made of filter paper or similar material intended to be inserted under a patient's lower eyelid to stimulate and evaluate formation of tears.

***Schistosoma* spp. Serological Reagents** Class I devices that consist of antigens and antisera used in serological tests to identify *Schistosoma* spp. antibodies in a patient's serum. The identification aids in the diagnosis of schistosomiasis caused by parasitic flatworms of the genus *Schistosoma*. Schistosomiasis is characterized by a variety of acute and chronic infections. Acute infection is marked by fever, allergic symptoms and diarrhea. Chronic effects are usually severe and are caused by fibrous degeneration of tissue around deposited eggs of the parasite in the liver, lungs, and central nervous system. Schistosomes can also cause schistosome dermatitis (e.g., swimmer's itch) a skin disease marked by intense itching.

Scintillation (Gamma) Camera   A Class I device intended to image the distribution of radionuclides in the body by means of a photon radiation detector. This generic type of device may include signal analysis and display equipment, patient and equipment supports, radionuclide anatomical markers, component parts, and accessories.

Scissors (Surgical tissue)   A Class I device used to cut soft tissue of the mouth, such as gums, during surgical procedures. The device has short, slightly curved stainless steel blades which allow easy access to the surgical site.

Scleral Shell   A Class II device made of glass or plastic that is intended to be inserted for short time periods over the cornea and proximal cornea sclera for cosmetic or reconstructive purposes. An artificial eye is usually painted on the device. The device is not intended to be implanted.

Selective Culture Medium   A Class I device that consists primarily of liquid and/or solid biological materials used to cultivate and identify certain microorganisms. The device contains one or more components that suppress the growth of certain microorganisms while either promoting or not affecting the growth of other microorganisms. The device aids in the diagnosis of disease caused by pathogenic microorganisms and also provides epidemiological information on these diseases.

Seminal Fluid (Sperm) Immunological Test System   A Class I device that consists of the reagents used, for legal purposes, to identify and differentiate animal and human semen. The test results can be used as court evidence in alleged instances of rape and other sex-related crimes.

***Serratia* spp. Serological Reagents**   Class I devices that consist of antigens and antisera used in serological tests to identity *Serratia* spp. from cultured isolates derived from clinical specimens. The identification aids in the diagnosis of disease caused by bacteria belonging to the genus *Serratia* and provides epidemiological information on these diseases. *Serratia* spp. are occasionally associated with gastroenteritis (food poisoning) and wound infections.

Set (Audiometer calibration set)   An electronic reference Class II device that is intended to calibrate an audiometer. It measures the sound frequency and intensity characteristics that emanate from an audiometer earphone. The device consists of an acoustic cavity of known volume, a sound level meter, a microphone with calibration traceable to the National Bureau of Standards, oscillators, frequency counters, microphone amplifiers, and a recorder. The device can measure selected audiometer test frequencies at a given intensity level, and selectable audiometer attenuation settings at a given test frequency.

Shigella spp. Serological Reagents Class II devices that consist of antigens and antisera including antisera conjugated with a fluorescent dye (immunofluorescent reagents) used in serological tests to identify *Shigella* spp. from cultured isolates. The identification aids in the diagnosis of shigellosis caused by bacteria belonging to the genus *Shigella* and provides epidemiological information on this disease. *Shigellosis* is characterized by abdominal pain, cramps, diarrhea, and fever.

Short Increment Sensitivity Index (SISI) Adapter A Class I device used with an audiometer in diagnostic hearing evaluations. An SISI adapter provides short, periodic, sound pulses in specific small decibel increments that are intended to be superimposed on the audiometer's output tone frequency.

Shortwave Diathermy A Class II device for use in applying therapeutic deep heat. It is a device that applies the electromagnetic energy of pulsed and/or continuous radiowaves in the radiofrequency bands of 13–27.12 megahertz to provide therapeutic deep heat in specific areas of the body. Such tissue heating is used as adjunctive therapy for the relief of pain in selected medical conditions, such as muscle spasms and joint contractures.

Shoulder Joint Glenoid (Hemi-shoulder) Metallic Cemented Prosthesis A Class III device that has a glenoid (socket) component made of alloys such as cobalt-chromium-molybdenum, or alloys with ultra-high molecular weight polyethylene, and intended to be implanted to replace part of a shoulder joint. This generic type of device is limited to those prostheses intended for use with bone cement.

Shoulder Joint Humeral (Hemi-shoulder) Metallic Uncemented Prosthesis A Class II device made of alloys such as cobalt-chromium-molybdenum. It has an intramedullary stem and is intended to be implanted to replace the articular surface of the proximal end of the humerus and to be fixed without bone cement. This device is not intended for biological fixation.

Shoulder Joint Metal/Metal or Metal/Polymer Constrained Cemented Prosthesis A Class III device intended to be implanted to replace a shoulder joint. The device prevents dislocation in more than one anatomic plane and has components that are linked together. This generic type of device includes prostheses that have a humeral component made of alloys, such as cobalt-chromium-molybdenum, and a glenoid component made of this alloy or a combination of this alloy and ultra-high molecular weight polyethylene. This generic type of device is limited to those prostheses intended for use with bone cement.

Shoulder Joint Metal/Polymer Nonconstrained Cemented Prosthesis A Class III device intended to be implanted to replace a shoulder joint. The device limits minimally (less than normal anatomic constraints) translation in one or more planes. It has no linkage across-the-joint. This generic type of device includes prostheses that have a humeral component made of alloys, such as cobalt-chromium-molybdenum, and a glenoid resurfacing component made of ultra-high molecular weight polyethylene, and is limited to those prostheses intended for use with bone cement.

Shoulder Joint Metal/Polymer Semiconstrained Cemented Prosthesis A Class III device intended to be implanted to replace a shoulder joint. The device limits translation and rotation in one or more planes via the geometry of its articulating surfaces. It has no linkage across-the-joint. This generic type of device includes prostheses that have a humeral resurfacing component made of alloys, such as cobalt-chromium-molybdenum, and a glenoid resurfacing component made of ultra-high molecular weight polyethylene, and is limited to those prostheses intended for use with bone cement.

Shunt (Endolymphatic shunt) A Class II device that consists of a tube or sheet intended to be implanted to relieve the symptoms of vertigo. The device permits the unrestricted flow of excess endolymph from the distended end of the endolymphatic system into the mastoid cavity where resorption occurs. This device is made of polytetrafluoroethylene or silicone elastomer.

Shunt (Endolymphatic shunt tube with valve) A Class III device that consists of a pressure-limiting valve associated with a tube intended to be implanted in the inner ear to relieve the symptoms of vertigo. The device directs excess endolymph from the distended end of the endolymphatic system into the mastoid cavity where resorption occurs. The function of the pressure-limiting, inner ear valve is to impede the flow of endolymph so that a physiologically normal endolymphatic pressure is maintained. The device is made of silicone elastomer and polyamide and contains gold radiopaque markers within the silicone elastomer sheath.

Sickle Cell Test A Class II device used to determine the sickle cell hemoglobin content of human blood to detect sickle cell anemia (a hereditary hemolytic anemia characterized by joint and abdominal pain, leg ulcers, and sickle-shaped erythrocytes).

Signal Isolation System A Class II device that electrically isolates the patient from equipment connected to the domestic power system. This isolation may be accomplished, for example, by transformer coupling, acoustic coupling, or optical coupling.

Silicate Protector A Class I device made of silicone that is applied with an absorbent tipped applicator to the surface of a new restoration to temporarily exclude fluids from its surface.

Silicone Gel-Filled Breast Prosthesis Class III devices made of: (1) Single-lumen silicone gel-filled breast prosthesis. A single-lumen silicone gel-filled breast prosthesis is a silicone rubber shell made of polysiloxane(s), such as polydimethylsiloxane and poly-diphenylsiloxane. The shell either contains a fixed amount cross-linked polymerized silicone gel, filler, and stabilizers or is filled to the desired size with injectable silicone gel at time of implantation. The device is intended to be implanted to augment or reconstruct the female breast. (2) Double-lumen silicone gel-filled breast pros-thesis. A double lumen silicone gel-filled breast prosthesis is a sili-cone rubber inner shell and a silicone rubber outer shell. Both shells are made of polysiloxane(s), such as polydimethylsiloxane and polydiphenylsiloxane. The inner shell contains fixed amounts of cross-linked polymerized silicone gel, fillers, and stabilizers. The outer shell is inflated to the desired size with sterile isotonic saline before or after implantation. The device is intended to be implanted to augment or reconstruct the female breast. (3) Polyurethane covered silicone gel-filled breast prosthesis. A polyurethane covered silicone gel-filled breast prosthesis is an inner silicone rub-ber shell made of polysiloxane(s), such as polydimethylsiloxane and polydiphenylsiloxane, with an outer silicone adhesive layer and an outer covering of polyurethane. Contained within the inner shell is a fixed amount of cross-linked polymerized silicone gel, fillers, and stabilizers and an inert support structure compartmen-talizing the silicone gel. The device is intended to be implanted to augment or reconstruct the female breast. Note: Date premarket ap-proval application (PMA) is required. A PMA is required to be filed with the Food and Drug Administration on or before July 9, 1991, for any silicone gel-filled breast prosthesis that was in commercial dis-tribution before May 28, 1976, or that has, on or before July 9, 1991, been found to be substantially equivalent to a silicone gel-filled breast prosthesis that was in commercial distribution before May 28, 1976. Any other silicone gel-filled breast prosthesis shall have an approved PMA in effect before being placed in commercial distribu-tion.

Silicone Inflatable Breast Prosthesis   A Class III device composed of a silicone rubber shell made of polysiloxane(s), such as poly-dimethylsiloxane and polydiphenylsiloxane, that is inflated to the desired size with sterile isotonic saline before or after implantation. The device is intended to be implanted to augment or reconstruct the female breast.

Simulatan (Including crossed cylinder)   A Class I device that is a set of pairs of cylinder lenses that provides various equal plus and minus refractive strengths. The lenses are arranged so that the user can exchange the positions of plus and minus cylinder lenses of equal strengths. The device is intended for subjective refraction (refraction in which the patient judges whether a given object is clearly in focus as the examiner uses different lenses).

Single/Multiple Component Metallic Bone Fixation Appliances and Accessories   Class II devices intended to be implanted and consist-ing of one or more metallic components and their metallic fasteners.

The devices contain a plate, a nail/plate combination, or a blade/plate combination that are made of alloys, such as cobalt-chromium-molybdenum, stainless steel, and titanium, that are intended to be held in position with fasteners, such as screws and nails, or bolts, nuts, and washers. These devices are used for fixation of fractures of the proximal or distal end of long bones, such as intracapsular, intertrochanteric, intercervical, supracondylar, or condylar fractures of the femur; for fusion of a splint; or for surgical procedures that involve cutting a bone. The devices may be implanted or attached through the skin so that a pulling force (traction) may be applied to the skeletal system.

Skiascopic Rack A Class II device that is a rack and a set of attached ophthalmic lenses of various dioptric strengths intended as an aid in refraction.

Skin Marker A pen-like Class I device intended to be used to write on the patient's skin, e.g., to outline surgical incision sites or mark anatomical sites for accurate blood pressure measurement.

Smooth or Threaded Metallic Bone Fixation Fastener A Class II device intended to be implanted that consists of a stiff wire segment or rod made of alloys, such as cobalt-chromium-molybdenum and stainless steel, and that may be smooth on the outside, fully or partially threaded, straight, or U-shaped. It may be either blunt pointed, sharp pointed, or have a formed, slotted head on the end. It may be used for fixation of bone fractures, for bone reconstructions, as a guide pin for insertion of other implants, or it may be implanted through the skin so that a pulling force (traction) may be applied to the skeletal system.

Sodium Test System A Class II device intended to measure sodium in serum, plasma, and urine. Measurements obtained by this device are used in the diagnosis and treatment of aldosteronism (excessive secretion of the hormone aldosterone), diabetes insipidus (chronic excretion of large amounts of dilute urine accompanied by extreme thirst), adrenal hypertension, Addison's disease (caused by destruction of the adrenal glands), dehydration, inappropriate antidiuretic hormone secretion, or other diseases involving electrolyte imbalance.

Soft (Hydrophilic) Contact Lens A Class III device intended to be worn directly against the cornea and adjacent limbal and scleral areas of the eye to correct vision conditions or act as a therapeutic bandage. The device is made of various polymer materials, the main polymer molecules of which absorb or attract a certain volume (percentage) of water.

Soft (Hydrophilic) Contact Lens Solution A Class III device intended to clean, disinfect, wet, or store a soft (hydrophilic) contact.

Solvent (Surgical skin degreaser or adhesive tape solvent) A Class

I device that consists of a liquid, such as 1,1,2-trichloro-1,2,2-trifluoroethane; 1,1,1-trichloroethane; and 1,1,1-trichloroethane with mineral spirits, intended to be used to dissolve surface skin oil or adhesive tape.

Sonic Surgical Instrument and Accessories/Attachments A hand-held Class II device with various accessories or attachments, such as a cutting tip that vibrates at high frequencies, and is intended for medical purposes to cut bone or other materials, such as acrylic.

Sorbitol Dehydrogenase Test System A Class I device intended to measure the activity of the enzyme sorbitol dehydrogenase in serum. Measurements obtained by this device are used in the diagnosis and treatment of liver disorders such as cirrhosis or acute hepatitis.

Special Grade Wheelchair A Class II device with wheels that provides mobility for those persons restricted to a sitting position and that is designed for long-term use in all environments (e.g., for paraplegics, quadraplegics, and amputees).

Specimen Collection and Transport Device A Class I device that is a sterile specimen collecting chamber that preserves the viability of microorganisms during storage following collection and transport from the specimen collecting area to the laboratory. The device aids in the diagnosis of disease caused by pathogenic microorganisms and also provides epidemiological information on these diseases.

Specimen Transport and Storage Container A Class I device used to contain biological specimens during storage and transport within and between clinics and laboratories in such an environment that the specimen can effectively be used for histological or cytological examination.

Spectacle Dissociation Test System An AC-powered or battery-powered Class I device, such as Lancaster test system, that consists of a light source and various filters, usually red or green filters, intended to subjectively measure imbalance of ocular muscles.

Spectacle Frame A Class I device made of metal or plastic intended to hold prescription spectacle lenses worn by a patient to correct refractive errors.

Speculum and Accessories A Class I device intended to be inserted into a body cavity to aid observation. It is either nonilluminated or illuminated and may have various accessories.

Spinal Fluid Pressure Manometer A Class II device used to measure the spinal fluid pressure. The device uses a hollow needle, which is inserted into the spinal column fluid space, to connect the spinal fluid to a graduated column so that the pressure can be measured by reading the height of the fluid.

Spinal Interlaminal Fixation Orthosis   A Class II device intended to be implanted made of an alloy, such as stainless steel, that consists of various hooks and a posteriorly placed compression or distraction rod. The device is implanted, usually across three adjacent vertebrae, to straighten and immobilize the spine to allow bone grafts in order to unite and fuse the vertebrae together. The device is used primarily in the treatment of scoliosis (a lateral curvature of the spine), but it also may be used in the treatment of fracture or dislocation of the spine, grades 3 and 4 of spondylolisthesis (a dislocation of the spinal column), and lower back syndrome.

Spinal Intervertebral Body Fixation Orthosis   A Class II device intended to be implanted that is made of titanium. It consists of various vertebral plates that are punched into each of a series of vertebral bodies. An eye-type screw is inserted in a hole in the center of each of the plates. A braided cable is threaded through each eye-type screw. The cable is tightened with a tension device and it is fastened or crimped at each eye-type screw. The device is used to apply force to a series of vertebrae to correct "sway back" scoliosis (lateral curvature of the spine), or other spinal conditions.

Spirometer, Diagnostic   A Class II device used in pulmonary function testing to measure the volume of gas moving in and out of the lungs.

Spirometer, Monitoring   A Class II device used to continuously measure tidal volume (volume of gas inhaled during each respiration cycle), or minute volume (tidal volume multiplied by the rate of respiration for one minute) for evaluation of ventilatory status.

***Sporothrix schenckii* Serological Reagents**   Class I devices that consist of antigens and antisera used in serological tests to identify *Sporothrix schenckii* antibodies in a patient's serum.

Spot-Film Device   A Class II device that is an electromechanical component of a fluoroscopic X-ray system that is intended to be used for medical purposes to position a radiographic film cassette to obtain radiographs during fluoroscopy.

Spring-Powered Jet Injector   A Class II device consisting of a syringe used to administer a local anesthetic. The syringe is powered by a spring mechanism that provides the pressure to force the anesthetic out of the syringe.

Stabilized Enzyme Solution   A Class II device composed of a reagent used to enhance the reactivity of red blood cells with certain antibodies, including antibodies that are not detectable by other techniques. These enzyme solutions include papain, bromelin, ficin, and trypsin.

Stair-Climbing Wheelchair   A mobility assist Class III device used by a disabled person to climb stairs in a sitting position. The device functions by means of two endless belt tracks that are lowered from under the chair and adjusted to the angle of the stairs.

Stand-On Patient Scale   A Class I device used to weigh a patient who is able to stand on the scale platform.

Stand-Up Wheelchair   A "heeled mobility" Class II assist device that also operates as an external manually controlled mechanical system that enables a paraplegic to stand by means of an elevating seat.

Staphylococcal Typing Bacteriophage   A Class I device consisting of a bacterial virus used to identify pathogenic staphylococcal bacteria through use of this bacteria's susceptibility to cell destruction by the virus. Test results are used principally for the collection of epidemiological information.

***Staphylococcus aureus* Serological Reagents**   Class I devices that consist of antigens and antisera used in serological tests to identify enterotoxin (toxin affecting the intestine) producing staphylococci from cultured isolates derived from food sources. The identification aids in the diagnosis of disease caused by this bacteria belonging to the genus *Staphylococcus* and provides epidemiological information on these diseases. Certain strains of *Staphylococcus aureus* produce an enterotoxin while growing in meat, dairy, or bakery products. After ingestion this enterotoxin is absorbed in the gut and causes destruction of the intestinal lining (gastroenteritis).

Staple (Implantable staple)   A staple-like Class II device intended to connect internal tissues to aid healing. It is not absorbable.

Staple (Removable skin staple)   A staple-like Class I device intended to connect external tissues temporarily to aid healing. It is not absorbable.

Stationary X-ray System   A Class II device that is a permanently installed diagnostic system intended to generate and control X-rays for examination of various anatomical regions. This generic type of device may include signal analysis and display equipment, patient and equipment supports, component parts, and accessories.

Statute	Purpose	Regulation
510	Good Laboratory Practices	21 CFR 58
510(k)	Premarket Notification	21 CFR 807
514	Voluntary Standards	21 CFR 861
515	Premarket Approval	21 CFR 814
518	Recall	21 CFR 7
519	Records and Reports	21 CFR 803
520(f)	Good Manufacturing Pract.	21 CFR 820
520 (g)	Invest. Dev. Exemption	21 CFR 812.27
		21 CFR 813 812.25(d)
		21 CFR 50 and 56
726	Color Additives	21 CFR 70 and 73

Stent, Ureteral A Class II implantable device that is a catheter (stent) inserted into the ureter to provide ureteral rigidity and allow the unimpeded passage of urine. The device may have distal protrusions or hooked ends to keep the device in place during treatment of ureteral injuries and obstructions.

Stereoscope An AC-powered or battery-powered Class I device that combines the images of two similar objects to produce a three-dimensional appearance of solidity and relief. It is intended to measure the angle of strabismus (eye muscle deviation), evaluate binocular vision (usage of both eyes to see), and guide a patient's corrective exercises of eye muscles.

Sterilization Indicator A Class II device used to show, by visible or measurable evidence, that a treated medical product was sufficiently exposed to a sterilization agent to allow the user to assume that the product is sterile.

Steriopsis Measuring Instrument A Class I device intended to measure depth perception by illumination of objects placed on different planes.

Stethoscope A Class I device that mechanically or electrically amplifies sounds associated with the heart, arteries, and veins.

Stethoscope Head A Class I diagnostic anesthesiology device comprising a weighed chest piece used during anesthesia to listen to the heart, breathing, and other physiological sounds.

Stimulator A Class II device that applies electrical current to a nerve to treat certain chronic conditions.

Stimulator (Electrical peripheral nerve stimulator) A Class II device (peripheral nerve stimulator or neuromuscular blockade monitor) used to apply an electrical current to a patient to test the level of pharmacological effect of anesthetic drugs and gases.

Stimulator, Cranial Electrotherapy A Class III device intended to provide electrical stimulation to a patient's head to treat insomnia, depression, or anxiety.

Stimulator, Diaphragmatic/Phrenic Nerve A Class III implantable device that provides electrical stimulation to the phrenic nerve and produces normal breathing during hypoventilation (a state in which an abnormally low amount of air enters the lungs), which is caused by brain stem disease, high cervical spinal cord injury, or chronic lung disease. The stimulator consists of an implanted receiver with electrodes placed around the phrenic nerve and an external transmitter for stimulating pulses across the skin to the implanted receiver.

Stimulator, Diaphragmatic/Subcortical Nerve A Class III implantable device that applies electrical current to subsurface areas of the brain to treat severe intractable pain. The stimulator consists of an implantable receiver with electrodes placed within the brain, and an external transmitter for the stimulating pulses across the skin to the implanted receiver.

Stimulator, Neuromuscular A Class II implantable device that provides electrical stimulation to the peroneal or femoral nerve causing muscle contraction, thus improving the gait in a paralyzed leg. The stimulator consists of an implanted receiver with electrodes placed around the nerve, and an external transmitter for the stimulating pulses across the skin. The external transmitter is activated by a switch in the heel of the patient's shoe.

Stimulator, Spinal Cord A Class III implantable device used to help in emptying the bladders of paraplegics with complete transection of the spinal cord, who are unable to empty their bladders by reflex means or by intermittent use of catheters. The device consists of an implanted receiver with electrodes placed on the conus medullaris, and an external transmitter for stimulating pulses across the skin to the implanted receiver.

Stomach pH Electrode A Class II device used to measure intragastric and intraesophageal pH (hydrogen ion concentration). The pH electrode is at the end of a flexible lead that may be inserted into the stomach through the patient's mouth and esophagus. The device may include an integral gastrointestinal tube.

***Streptococcus* spp. Exoenzyme Reagents** Class II devices used in serological tests to identify *Streptococcus* spp. exoenzyme antibodies in a patient's serum. The identification aids in the diagnosis of disease caused by bacteria belonging to the genus *Streptococcus* and provides epidemiological information on these diseases. Pathogenic streptococci are associated with infections such as sore throat, impetigo (an infection characterized by small pustules on the skin), urinary tract infections, rheumatic fever, and kidney disease.

***Streptococcus* spp. Serological Reagents** Class I devices that consist of antigens and antisera (excluding streptococcal exoenzyme reagents made from enzymes secreted by streptococci spp. used in serological tests to identify streptococcus spp. from cultured isolates derived from clinical specimens. The identification aids in the diagnosis of diseases caused by bacteria belonging to the genus *Streptococcus* and provides epidemiological information on these diseases. Pathogenic streptococci are associated with infections, such as sore throat, impetigo (an infection characterized by small pustules on the skin), and urinary tract infections; with allergic-type reactions, such as rheumatic fever and kidney disease.

Suction Antichoke Device A Class III device intended to be used in an emergency situation to remove, by the application of suction, foreign objects that obstruct a patient's airway in order to prevent asphyxiation of the patient.

Sulfhemoglobin Assay A Class II device consisting of the reagents, calibrators, controls, and instrumentation used to determine the sulfhemoglobin (a compound of sulfur and hemoglobin) content of human blood as an aid in the diagnosis of sulfhemoglobinemia (presence of sulfhemoglobin in the blood due to drug administration or exposure to a poison). This measurement may be made using methods such as spectroscopy, colorimetry, spectrophotometry, and gasometry.

Sulfonamide Test System A Class I device intended to measure sulfonamides, any of the antibacterial drugs derived from sulfanilamide, in human specimens. Measurements obtained by this device are used in the diagnosis and treatment of sulfonamide overdose, and in monitoring sulfonamide levels to ensure appropriate therapy.

Sunglasses (Nonprescription) Class I devices that consist of spectacle frames or clips with absorbing, reflective, tinted, polarizing, or photosensitized lenses intended to be worn by a person to protect the eyes from bright sunlight, but not to provide refractive corrections. This device is usually available over-the-counter.

Supplement for Culture Media A Class I device, such as a vitamin or sugar mixture, that is added to a solid or liquid basal culture medium to produce a desired formulation and that is used to enhance the growth of fastidious microorganisms (having complex nutritional requirements). This device aids in the diagnosis of diseases caused by pathogenic microorganisms.

Support Gel for Clinical Use A Class I device that consists of an agar or agarose preparation that is used while measuring various kinds of or parts of protein molecules by various immunochemical techniques, such as immunoelectrophoresis, immunodiffusion or chromatography.

Surgeon's Glove A Class I device made of natural or synthetic rubber intended to be worn by operating room personnel to protect a surgical wound from contamination. The lubricating or dusting powder used in the glove is excluded.

Surgeon's Gloving Cream A Class I device composed of an ointment intended to by used to lubricate the user's hand before putting on a surgeon's glove.

Surgical Apparel Class II devices that are intended to be worn by operating room personnel during surgical procedures to protect both the surgical patient and the operating room personnel from transfer of microorganisms, body fluids, and particulate material. Examples include surgical caps, hoods, masks, gowns, operating room shoes and shoe covers, and isolation masks and gowns. Surgical suits and dresses, commonly known as scrub suits, are excluded. Note: Class II for surgical gowns and surgical masks. Class I for surgical apparel other than surgical gowns and surgical masks.

Surgical Camera and Accessories A Class I device intended to be used to record operative procedures.

Surgical Drape and Drape Accessories A Class II device made of natural or synthetic materials intended to be used as a protective patient covering, such as to isolate a site of surgical incision from microbial and other contamination. The device includes a plastic wound protector that may adhere to the skin around a surgical incision or be placed in a wound to cover its exposed edges, and a latex drape with a self-retaining finger cot that is intended to allow repeated insertion of the surgeon's finger into the rectum during performance of a transurethral prostatectomy.

Surgical Headlight A Class I device that is attached to the user's head and used as a supplementary or auxiliary light source to illuminate the oral cavity during surgical procedures.

Surgical Instrument Motors and Accessories/Attachments AC-powered, battery-powered, or air-powered Class I devices intended for use during surgical procedures to provide power to operate various accessories or attachments in order to cut hard tissue or bone and soft tissue. Accessories or attachments may include a bur, chisel (osteotome), dermabrasion brush, dermatome, drill bit, hammerhead, pin driver, and saw blade.

Surgical Lamp (Including a fixture) A Class II device intended to be used to provide visible illumination of the surgical field or the patient.

Surgical Mesh A Class II device made of a metallic or polymeric screen intended to be implanted to reinforce soft tissue or bone where weakness exists. Examples of surgical mesh are metallic and polymeric mesh for hernia repair, and acetabular and cement restrictor mesh used during orthopedic surgery.

Surgical Microscope and Accessories An AC-powered Class I device intended for use during surgery to provide a magnified view of the surgical field.

Surgical Nerve Stimulator/Locator A Class II device that is intended to provide electrical stimulation to the body to locate and identify nerves and to test their excitability.

Surgical Reconstruction A repair to immobilize maxillofacial bone fragments in their proper facial relationship.

Surgical Skin Degreaser or Adhesive Tape Solvent A Class I device that consists of a liquid, such as 1,1,2-trichloro-1,2,2-trifluoroethane; 1,1,1-trichloroethane; and 1,1,1-trichloroethane with mineral spirits intended to be used to dissolve surface skin oil or adhesive tape.

Surgical Sponge Scale A surgical sponge scale is a nonelectrically powered Class I device used to weigh surgical sponges that have been used to absorb blood during surgery so that, by comparison with the known dry weight of the sponges, an estimate may be made of the blood lost by a patient during surgery.

Surgical Tissue Scissors A Class I device used to cut soft tissue of the mouth, such as gums, during surgical procedures. The device has short, slightly curved stainless steel blades that allow easy access to the surgical site.

Surgical Vessel Dilator A Class II device used to enlarge or calibrate a vessel.

Suture (Absorbable poly[glycolide/L-lactide] surgical suture) A Class II device composed of an absorbable sterile, flexible strand as prepared and synthesized from homopolymers of glycolide and copolymers made from 90 percent glycolide and 10 percent lactide, and is indicated for use in soft tissue approximation. A PGL suture meets *United States Pharmacopeia* (U.S.P.) requirements as described in the U.S.P. *Monograph for Absorbable Surgical Sutures*. It may be monofilament or multifilament (braided) in form; it may be uncoated or coated; it may be undyed or dyed with an FDA-approved color additive. Also, the suture may be provided with or without a standard needle attached.

Suture (Absorbable surgical gut suture) A Class II device both plain and chromic, composed of an absorbable, sterile, flexible thread prepared from either the serosal connective tissue layer of beef (bovine), or the submucosal fibrous tissue of sheep (ovine) intestine, and is intended for use in soft tissue approximation.

Suture (Nonabsorbable polyamide surgical suture) A nonabsorbable, sterile, Class II device made of a flexible thread prepared from long-chain aliphatic polymers Nylon 6 and Nylon 6,6 and is indicated for use in soft tissue approximation. The polyamide surgical suture meets *United States Pharmacopeia* (U.S.P.) requirements as described in the U.S.P. *Monograph for Nonabsorbable Surgical Sutures*. It may be monofilament of multifilament in form, uncoated or coated, undyed or dyed with an appropriate FDA listed color additive. Also, the suture may be provided with or without a standard needle attached.

Suture (Nonabsorbable poly(ethylene terephthalate) surgical suture) A multifilament, nonabsorbable, sterile, flexible thread Class II device prepared from fibers of high molecular weight, long-chain, linear polyesters having recurrent aromatic rings as an integral component and is indicated for use in soft tissue approximation. The poly(ethylene terephthalate) surgical suture meets U.S.P. requirements as described in the U.S.P. *Monograph for Nonabsorbable Surgical Sutures*. It may be provided uncoated or coated, undyed or dyed with an appropriate FDA listed color additive. Also,

187

the suture may be provided with or without a standard needle attached.

Suture (Nonabsorbable polypropylene surgical suture)   A monofilament, nonabsorbable, sterile flexible Class II device composed of a thread prepared from long-chain polyolefin polymer known as polypropylene and is indicated for use in soft tissue approximation. The polypropylene surgical suture meets *United States Pharmacopeia* (U.S.P.) requirements as described in the U.S.P. *Monograph for Nonabsorbable Surgical Sutures.* It may be undyed or dyed with an FDA approved color additive, and the suture may be provided with or without a standard needle attached.

Suture Retention Device   A Class I device, such as a retention bridge, a surgical button, or a suture bolster, intended to aid wound healing by distributing suture tension over a larger area in the patient.

Switching Valve   A Class I diagnostic anesthesiology device comprising a three-way valve located between a stethoscope placed over the heart, a blood presure cuff, and an earpiece. The valve allows the user to eliminate one sound channel and listen to only heart or Korotoff (blood pressure) sounds through the other channel.

Synthetic Cell and Tissue Culture Media and Components   Class I devices made of substances that are composed entirely of defined components (e.g., amino acids, vitamins, inorganic salts, etc.) that are essential for the survival and development of cell lines of humans and other animals.

Syringe (Periodontic or endodontic irrigating)   A Class I device used for the irrigation of tissues in the mouth, such as gums in periodontic therapy and root canals in teeth in endodontic therapy.

Syringe (Restorative or impression material)   A Class I device used in the placement of impression material (alginate) or restorative material (amalgam) in the oral cavity. It consists of a hollow tube syringe body with a plunger at one end and a narrow opening at the opposite end, through which the impression or restorative material is forced by the plunger.

Syringe Actuator for Injectors   A Class II device that electrically controls the timing of an injection by an angiographic or indicator injector and synchronizes the injection with the electrocardiograph (ECG) signal.

System for the Identification of Hepatitis B Antigen   A Class I device that consists of the equipment and reagents necessary for the detection of hepatitis B antigen. Hepatitis B antigen is usually detected by radioimmunoassay, reversed passive hemagglutination, counterelectrophoresis, or latex agglutination. The device does not include articles that are licensed by the Bureau of Biologics of the Food and Drug Administration.

Systemic Lupus Erythematosus Immunological Test System A Class II device that consists of the reagents used to measure, by immunochemical techniques, the autoimmune antibodies in serum and body fluids that react with cellular nuclear double-stranded deoxyribonucleic acid (DNA) or other nuclear constituents that are specifically diagnostic of SLE. Measurement of nuclear double-stranded DNA antibodies aids in the diagnosis of systemic lupus erythematosus (a multisystem autoimmune disease in which tissues are attacked by the person's own antibodies).

T

Table (Manual operating table and accessories and manual operating chair and accessories) Nonpowered Class I devices, usually with movable components, intended to be used to support a patient during diagnostic examinations or surgical procedures.

Table (Operating tables and accessories and operating chairs and accessories) AC-powered or air-powered Class I devices, usually with movable components, intended for use during diagnostic examinations or surgical procedures to support and position a patient.

Tangent Screen (Campimeter) An AC-powered or battery-powered Class I device that is a large, square, cloth chart with a central mark of fixation intended to map on a flat surface the central 30° of a patient's visual field. This generic type of device includes projection tangent screens, target tangent screens and targets, felt tangent screens, and stereo campimeters.

Tee Drain (Water tap) A Class II device that traps and drains water that collects in a ventilator tubing during respiratory therapy, thereby preventing an increase in breathing resistance.

Teething Ring A Class I soft plastic device containing a liquid, such as water. Prior to use, the liquid may be chilled by refrigerating the device. The device is used by infants to soothe gums during the teething process.

Telephone Electrocardiograph (Transmitters and receivers) A Class II device used to condition an ECG signal so that it can be transmitted via telephone to another location. This device also includes a receiver that reconditions the received signal into its original format so that it can be displayed. This device includes other devices used to transmit and receive pacemaker signals.

Template for Clinical Use A Class I device that consists of a pattern or guide intended for medical purposes, such as selecting or positioning orthopedic implants or guiding the marking of tissue before cutting.

Temporary Crown and Bridge Resin A Class II device composed of a material, such as polymethylmethacrylate, that is used to make a temporary prosthesis such as a crown or bridge. The temporary prosthesis is used until a permanent restoration is fabricated.

Test System (α-1-Antichymotrypsin immunological test system) A Class II device that consists of the reagents used to measure, by immunochemical techniques, α-1-antichymotrypsin (a protein) in serum, tissues, and body fluids. α-1-Antichymotrypsin helps protect tissues against proteolytic (protein-splitting) enzymes released during infection.

Test System (Antimitochondrial antibody immunological test system) A Class II device that consists of the reagents used to measure, by immunochemical techniques, antimitochondrial antibodies in human serum. The measurements aid in the diagnosis of diseases that produce a spectrum of autoantibodies (antibodies produced against the body's own tissue) such as primary biliary cirrhosis (degeneration of liver tissue) and chronic active hepatitis (inflammation of the liver).

Test System (Antinuclear antibody immunological test system) A Class II device that consists of the reagents used to measure, by immunochemical techniques, the autoimmune antibodies in serum and tissues that react with cellular nuclear constituents (molecules present in the nucleus of a cell, such as ribonucleic acid, deoxyribonucleic acid, or nuclear proteins) in serum or body fluids. The measurements aid in the diagnosis of systemic lupus erythematosus, a multisystem autoimmune disease (a disease in which antibodies attack the victim's own tissues), hepatitis (a liver disease), rheumatoid arthritis, Sjögren's syndrome (arthritis with inflammation of the eye, eyelid, and salivary glands), and systemic sclerosis (chronic hardening and shrinking of many body tissues).

Test System (Antiparietal antibody immunological test system) A Class II device that consists of the reagents used to measure, by immunochemical techniques, the specific antibody for gastric parietal cells in human serum and body fluids. Gastric parietal cells are those cells located in the stomach that produce a protein that enables vitamin B_{12} to be absorbed by the body. The measurements aid in the diagnosis of vitamin B_{12} deficiency (or pernicious anemia), atrophic gastritis (inflammation of the stomach), and autoimmune connective tissue diseases (diseases reculting when the body produces antibodies against its own tissues).

Test System (Antismooth muscle antibody immunological test system) A Class II device that consists of the reagents used to measure, by immunochemical techniques, the antismooth muscle antibodies (antibodies to nonstriated, involuntary muscle) in serum. The measurements aid in the diagnosis of chronic hepatitis (inflammation of the liver) and autoimmune connective tissue diseases (diseases resulting from antibodies produced against the body's own tissues).

Test System (α-Globulin immunological test system) A Class I device that consists of the reagents used to measure, by immunochemical techniques, the α-globulin (a serum protein) in serum and other body fluids. Measurements of α-globulin may aid in the diagnosis of inflammatory lesions, infections, severe burns, and a variety of other conditions.

Test System (α-1-Lipoprotein immunological test system) A Class II device that consists of the reagents used to measure, by immunochemical techniques, the α-1-lipoprotein (high density lipoprotein) in serum or plasma. Measurement of α-1-lipoprotein may aid in the diagnosis of Tangier's disease (a hereditary disorder of fat metabolism).

Test System (α-2-Macroglobulin Immunological Test System) A Class II device that consists of the reagents used to measure, by immunochemical techniques, the α-2-macroglobulin (a serum protein) in plasma. Measurement of α-2-macroglobulin may aid in the diagnosis of blood clotting or clot lysis disorders.

Tester (Auditory impedance tester) A Class II device that is intended to change the air pressure in the external auditory canal and measure and graph the mobility characteristics of the tympanic membrane to evaluate the functional condition of the middle ear. The device is used to determine abnormalities in the mobility of the tympanic membrane due to stiffness, flaccidity, or the presence of fluid in the middle ear cavity. The device is also used to measure the acoustic reflex threshold from contractions of the stapedial muscle, to monitor healing of tympanic membrane grafts or stapedectomies, or to monitor follow-up treatment for inflammation of the middle ear.

Testicular Prostheses A Class III device consisting of a solid or gel-filled, silicone rubber prosthesis that is implanted surgically to resemble a testicle.

Testing (Acoustic chamber for audiometric testing) A Class I device that is a room intended for use in conducting diagnostic hearing evaluations and that eliminates sound reflections and provides isolation from outside sounds.

Testing (Earphone cushion for audiometric testing) A Class I device that is used to cover an audiometer earphone during audiometric testing to provide an acoustic coupling (sound connection path) between the audiometer earphone and the patient's ear.

Testing (Electronic noise generator for audiometric testing) A Class II device that consists of a swept frequency generator, an amplifier, and an earphone. It is intended to introduce a masking noise into the nontest ear during an audiometric evaluation. The device minimizes the nontest ear's sensing of test tones and signals being generated for the ear being tested.

Testosterone Test System A Class I device intended to measure testosterone (a male sex hormone) in serum, plasma, and urine. Measurement of testosterone is used in the diagnosis and treatment of disorders involving the male sex hormones (androgens), including primary and secondary hypogonadism, delayed or precocious puberty, impotence in males and in females, hirsutism (excessive hair) and virilization (masculinization) due to tumors, polycystic ovaries, and adrenogenital syndromes.

Theophylline Test System A Class III device intended to measure theophylline (a drug used for stimulation of the muscles in the cardiovascular, respiratory, and central nervous systems) in serum and plasma. Measurements obtained by this device are used in the diagnosis and treatment of theophylline overdose or in monitoring levels of theophylline to ensure appropriate therapy.

Therapeutic Medical Binder A Class I device, usually made of cloth, that can be secured by ties so that it supports the underlying part of the body and/or holds a dressing in place.

Therapeutic Ultrasound and Muscle Stimulator A Class II device for use in applying therapeutic deep heat and muscle stimulation. It applies ultrasonic energy at a frequency beyond 20,000 cycles per second to provide therapeutic deep heat in specific areas of the body, and passes electrical currents through the affected body area to relax muscles. Such tissue heating and muscle stimulation is used as adjunctive therapy for the relief of pain in selected medical conditions such as muscle spasms and joint contractures.

Therapeutic X-ray Tube Housing Assembly A Class II device that is an X-ray generating tube encased in a radiation-shielded housing intended for use in radiation therapy. This generic type of device may include a high-voltage and filament transformers or other appropriate components when contained in radiation-shielded housing.

Thermal Cautery Unit An AC-powered or battery-powered Class II device intended for use during ocular surgery to coagulate tissue or arrest bleeding by heat conducted through a wire tip.

Thermal Regulating System A Class II device placed in contact with the patient and a temperature controller for the device. The system is used to regulate a patient's temperature.

Thermodilution Probe A Class II device that monitors cardiac output by use of thermodilution techniques. This device is commonly attached to a catheter that may have one or more probes.

Thermometer (Clinical color change) A Class II device used to measure oral or rectal body temperature by displaying the color changes of heat-sensitive liquid crystals. It is a disposable device with the liquid crystals (cholesteric esters) sealed in plastic at the end of a plastic strip.

Thermometer (Clinical electronic) A Class II device used to measure the body temperature of a patient by means of a transducer coupled with an electronic signal amplification, conditioning, and display unit. The transducer may be in a detechable probe with or without a disposable cover.

Thermometer (Clinical mercury) A Class II device used to measure oral, rectal, or axilllary body temperature using the thermal expansion of mercury.

Thin-Layer Chromatography (TLC) System for Clinical Use A Class I device intended to separate one or more drugs or compounds from a mixture. The mixture of compounds is absorbed onto a stationary phase or thin layer of inert material (e.g., cellulose, alumina, etc.) and eluted off by a moving solvent (moving phase) until equilibrium occurs between the two phases.

Thrombin Time Test A Class II device used to measure fibrinogen concentration and detect fibrin or fibrinogen split products for the evaluation of bleeding disorders.

Thromboplastin Generation Test A Class I device used to detect and identify coagulation factor deficiencies and coagulation inhibitors.

Thyroid Autoantibody Immunological Test System A Class II device that consists of the reagents used to measure, by immunochemical techniques, the autoantibodies (antibodies produced against the body's own tissues) to thyroid tissues. Measurement of thyroid autoantibodies may aid in the diagnosis of certain thyroid disorders, such as Hashimoto's disease (chronic lymphocytic thyroiditis), nontoxic goiter (enlargement of thyroid gland), Grave's disease (enlargement of the thyroid gland with protrusion of the eyeballs), and cancer of the thyroid.

Thyroid Stimulating Hormone Test System A Class II device intended to measure thyroid stimulating hormone, also known as thyrotrophin and thyrotrophic hormone, in serum and plasma. Measurements of thyroid stimulating hormone produced by the anterior pituitary are used in the diagnosis of thyroid or pituitary disorders.

Thyroxine-Binding Globulin Test System A Class II device intended to measure thyroxine (thyroid)-binding globulin (TBG), a plasma protein which binds thyroxine, in serum and plasma. Measurements obtained by this device are used in the diagnosis and treatment of thyroid diseases.

Tinnitus Masker An electronic Class III device intended to generate noise of sufficient intensity and bandwidth to mask ringing in the ears or internal head noises. Because the device is able to mask internal noises, it is also used as an aid in hearing external noises and speech.

Tissue Processing Equipment Class I devices used to prepare human tissue specimens for diagnostic histological examination by processing the specimens through the various stages of decalcifying, infiltrating, sectioning, and mounting on microscope slides. This device is also known as "decalcifying devices," "paraffin dispensers," "flotation baths," "infiltrators," "imbedding containers," "microtomes and accessories," "microscope slides and coverslips," and "slide-warming lamps and tables."

Titanium Subperiosteal Implant Material A Class II device composed of titanium that is used to construct custom prosthetic devices that are surgically implanted into the lower or upper jaw between the periosteum (connective tissue covering the bone) and supporting bony structures. The device provides support for prostheses such as dentures.

Tobramycin Test System A Class II device intended to measure tobramycin, an aminoglycoside antibiotic drug, in plasma and serum. Measurements obtained by this device are used in the diagnosis and treatment of tobramycin overdose and in monitoring levels of tobramycin to ensure appropriate therapy.

Toe Joint Phalangeal (Hemi-toe) Polymer Prosthesis A Class II device made of silicone elastomer intended to be implanted to replace the base of the proximal phalanx of the toe.

Toe Joint Polymer Constrained Prosthesis A Class II device made of silicone elastomer or polyester reinforced silicone elastomer intended to be implanted to replace the first metatarsophalangeal (big toe) joint. This generic type of device consists of a single flexible across-the-joint component that prevents dislocation in more than one anatomic plane.

Tomographic X-ray System An X-ray Class II device intended to be used to produce radiologic images of a specific cross-sectional plane of the body by blurring or eliminating detail from other planes. This generic type of device may include analysis and display equipment, patient and equipment supports, component parts, and accessories.

Tongs Antichoke Device A Class III device that is intended to be used in an emergency situation to grasp and remove foreign objects that obstruct a patient's airway in order to prevent asphyxiation of the patient. This generic type of device includes a plastic instrument with serrated ends that is inserted into the airway in a blind manner to grasp and extract foreign objects, and a stainless steel forceps with spoon ends that is inserted under tactile guidance to grasp and extract foreign objects from the airway.

Tonometer and Accessories A manual Class II device intended to measure intraocular pressure by applying a known force on the globe of the eye and measuring the amount of indentation produced (Schiotz type) or to measure intraocular tension by applanation (applying a small flat disk to the cornea). Accessories for the device may include a tonometer calibrator or a tonograph recording system. The device is intended for use in the diagnosis of glaucoma.

Tonometer Sterilizer An AC-powered Class I device intended to heat sterilize a tonometer (a device used to measure intraocular pressure).

Tooth Shade Resin Material A Class II device composed of materials such as bisphenol-A and glycidyl methacrylate (bis-GMA) that is used to restore carious lesions or structural defects in teeth.

Toothbrush (Manual) A Class I device intended to remove adherent plaque and food debris from the teeth to reduce tooth decay. It is composed of a shaft with either natural or synthetic bristles at one end.

Toothbrush (Powered) A Class I AC or battery-powered device intended to remove plaque or food particles from the teeth to reduce tooth decay. It consists of a handle containing a motor that provides vibrations to a toothbrush that is inserted in one end.

Topical Oxygen Chamber for Extremities A Class III device intended to hermetically surround a patient's limb and apply humidified oxygen topically at a pressure slightly greater than atmospheric pressure to aid healing of chronic skin ulcers or bed sores.

Total Ossicular Replacement Prosthesis A Class II device intended to be implanted for the total functional reconstruction of the ossicular chain, and facilitates the conduction of sound waves from the tympanic membrane to the inner ear. The device is made of materials such as polytetrafluoroethylene, polytetrafluoroethylene with vitreous carbon fiber composite, porous polyethylene, or from a combination of these materials.

Total Protein Test System A Class II device intended to measure total protein(s) in serum of plasma. Measurements obtained by this device are used in the diagnosis and treatment of a variety of diseases involving the liver, kidney, or bone marrow, as well as other metabolic or nutritional disorders.

Total Spinal Fluid Immunological Test System A Class I device that consists of the reagents used to measure, by immunochemical techniques, the total protein in cerebrospinal fluid. Measurement of spinal fluid proteins may aid in the diagnosis of inflammation of the central nervous system.

Total Thyroxine Test System A Class II device intended to measure total (free and protein bound) thyroxine (thyroid hormone) in serum and plasma. Measurements obtained by this device are used in the diagnosis and treatment of thyroid diseases.

Total Triiodothyronine Test System A Class II device intended to measure the hormone triiodothyronine in serum and plasma. Measurements obtained by this device are used in the diagnosis and treatment of thyroid diseases such as hyperthyroidism.

Tourniquet (Nonpneumatic tourniquet) A Class I device consisting of a strap or tubing intended to be wrapped around a patient's limb and tightened to reduce circulation.

Tourniquet (Pneumatic tourniquet) An air-powered Class II device consisting of a pressure-regulating unit, connecting tubing, and an inflatable cuff. The cuff is intended to be wrapped around a patient's limb and inflated to reduce or totally occlude circulation during surgery.

Toxoplasma gondii **Serological Reagents** Class II devices that consist of antigens and antisera used in serological tests to identify *Toxoplasma gondii* antibodies in a patient's serum. Additionally, some of these reagents consist of antisera conjugated with a fluorescent dye (immunofluorescent reagents) used to identify *Toxoplasma gondii* from clinical specimens. The identification aids in the diagnosis of toxoplasmosis caused by the parasitic protozoan *Toxoplasma gondii* and provides epidemiological information on this disease. Congenital toxoplasmosis is characterized by lesions of the central nervous system that, if undetected and untreated, may lead to brain defects, blindness, and death of an unborn fetus. The disease is characterized in children by inflammation of the brain and spinal cord.

Toynbee Diagnostic Tube A listening Class I device intended to determine the degree of openness of the eustachian tube.

Trace Microsphere A Class III device with trace nonbiodegradable microspheres.

Tracheal Prosthesis A tubular Class III device intended to be implanted to reconstruct the trachea.

Tracheal Tube A Class II device inserted into a patient's trachea via the nose or mouth and used to maintain an open airway.

Tracheal Tube Fixation Device A Class II device used to hold tracheal tubes in place, usually by means of straps or pinch rings.

Tracheal Tube Stylet A Class II device used to make a flexible tracheal tube rigid in order to facilitate intubation.

Tracheal/Bronchial Differential Ventilation Tube A Class II device used to isolate the left or right lung for anesthesia and pulmonary function testing.

Tracheobronchial Suction Catheter   A Class I device used to aspirate liquids or semisolids from a patient's upper airway.

Traction Accessories   Class I manual devices used with traction equipment to aid in exerting proper tensile (pulling) forces on the body. Examples of traction accessories are pulleys, straps, head halters, and pelvic restraints.

Transabdominal Amnioscope (Fetoscope) and Accessories   A Class III device designed to permit direct visual examination of the fetus by a telescopic system via abdominal entry. The device is used to ascertain fetal abnormalties, to obtain fetal blood samples, or to obtain fetal tissue. This generic type of device may include the following accessories: trocar and cannula, instruments used through an operating channel or through a separate cannula associated with the amnioscope, light source and cables, and component parts.

Transcervical Endoscope (Amnioscope) and Accessories   A Class II device designed to permit direct viewing of the fetus and amniotic sac by means of an open tube introduced into the uterus through the cervix. The device may be used to visualize the fetus or amniotic fluid and to sample fetal blood or amniotic fluid. This generic type of device may include obturators, instruments used through an operating channel, light sources and cables, and component parts.

Transcutaneous Electrical Nerve Stimulator (TENS)   A Class II device used for pain relief by applying an electrical current to electrodes fixed on the skin. The applied electric current is thought to prevent pain signals travelling in the nerves from reaching the brain.

Transducer   A Class II device used to measure pressure by converting mechanical inputs to electrical signals.

Transducer (Differential pressure)   A Class II two-chambered device used during pulmonary function testing. It generates an electrical signal for subsequent display or processing that is proportional to the difference in gas pressures in the two chambers.

Transducer, Apex Cardiographic   A Class II device used to detect motion of the heart (acceleration, velocity, or displacement) by changes in the mechanical or electrical properties of the device.

Transducer, Catheter Tip Pressure   A Class II device incorporated into the distal end of a catheter. When placed in the bloodstream, its mechanical or electrical properties change in relation to changes in blood pressure. These changes are in turn transmitted to accessory equipment for analysis.

197

Transducer, Extravascular Blood Pressure A Class II device used to measure blood pressure by changes in mechanical or electrical properties of the device. The proximal end of the transducer is connected to a pressure monitor that produces analog or digital electrical signals paralleling changes in blood pressure.

Transducer, Gas Flow A Class II device used to convert gas flow rate into an electrical signal for subsequent display or processing.

Transducer, Gas Pressure A Class II device used to convert gas pressure into an electrical signal for subsequent display or processing.

Transducer, Heart Sound A Class II device consisting of an external transducer that exhibits changes in mechanical or electrical properties in relation to cardiac sounds.

Transducer, Pressure A Class II device used to measure the pressure between a device and soft tissue by converting pressure inputs to analog electrical signals.

Transducer, Signal Amplifier and Signal Conditioner A Class II device used to provide the excitation energy for the transducer and to amplify or condition the signal emitted by the transmitter.

Transducer, Ultrasonic A Class II device applied to the skin to transmit and receive ultrasonic energy. It is used in conjunction with an echocardiograph as an aid in imaging cardiovascular structures. The device includes phased arrays and two-dimensional scanning transducers.

Transducer, Vessel Occlusion A Class II device used to supply an electrical signal corresponding to sounds produced in a partially occluded vessel. The device may include motion, sound, and ultrasonic transducers.

Transfer Set A Class I device composed of a piece of tubing with suitable adaptors used to transfer blood or plasma from one container to another.

Transilluminator An AC-powered or battery-powered Class I device that is a light source intended to transmit light through tissues to aid examination of patients.

Transmitter (Radiofrequency physiological signal and receivers) A Class II device used to condition a physiological signal so that it can be transmitted via radiofrequency from one location to another, e.g., a central monitoring station. The received signal is conditioned by the device into its original format so that it can be displayed.

Transmitter (Telephone electrocardiograph and receivers) A Class II device used to condition an ECG signal so that it can be transmitted via telephone to another location. This device also includes a receiver that reconditions the received signal into its original format so that it can be displayed. The device includes devices used to transmit and receive pacemaker signals.

Transport Culture Medium A Class I device that consists of a semi-solid, usually nonnutrient, medium that maintains the viability of suspected pathogens contained in patient specimens while in transit from the specimen collection area to the laboratory. The device aids in the diagnosis of disease caused by pathogenic microorganisms and also provides epidemiological information on these diseases.

Tray (Disposable fluoride) A Class I device made of styrofoam that is used for the topical application of fluoride to the teeth. To employ the tray, the patient bites down on the tray that has been filled with a fluoride solution.

Tray (Preformed impression) A Class I metal or plastic device used to hold impression material, such as alginate, during the making of an impression of a patient's teeth or alveolar process. The impression is used to reproduce the structure of a patient's teeth and gums.

***Treponema pallidum* Nontreponemal Test Reagents** Class II devices that consist of antigens and antisera that are derived from nontreponemal sources (sources not directly associated with treponemal organisms) and other control reagents (standardized reagents with which test results are compared). They are used to identify reagin, an antibody-like agent, that is produced from the reaction of treponemal microorganisms with certain body tissues. The identification aids in the diagnosis of syphilis, caused by bacteria belonging to the genus *Treponema*, and provides epidemiological information on syphilis. Syphilis is a contagious venereal disease that can lead to many structural skin-related lesions. It is transmitted by direct sexual contact or to a newborn by an infected mother (congenital syphilis).

***Treponema pallidum* Treponemal Test Reagents** Class II devices that consist of the antigens, antisera, and all control reagents (standardized reagents with which test results are compared) that are derived from treponemal sources. They are used in the fluorescent treponemal antibody absorption test (FTA-ABS), the *Treponema pallidum* immobilization test (T.P.I.), and other treponemal tests used to identify treponemal antibodies (antibodies induced directly from infecting treponemal organisms) in a patient's serum. The identification aids in the diagnosis of syphilis, caused by bacteria belonging to the genus *Treponema*, and provides epidemiological information on syphilis. Syphilis is a contagious venereal disease that can lead to many structural and skin-related lesions. It is transmitted either by direct sexual contact or to a newborn by an infected mother (congenital syphilis).

***Trichinella spiralis* Serological Reagents** Class I devices that consist of antigens and antisera used in serological tests to identify

199

Trichinella spiralis antibodies in a patient's serum. The identification aids in the diagnosis of trichinosis, caused by parasitic roundworms belonging to the genus *Trichinella*, and provides epidemiological information on trichinosis. Trichinosis is caused by ingestion of undercooked, infested meat, especially pork, and characterized by fever, muscle weakness, and diarrhea.

Tricyclic Antidepressant Drugs Test System A Class II device intended to measure any of the tricyclic antidepressant drugs in serum. The tricyclic antidepressant drugs include imipramine, desipramine, amitriptyline, nortriptyline, protriptyline, and doxepin. Measurements obtained by this device are used in the diagnosis and treatment of chronic depression to ensure appropriate therapy.

Triglyceride Test System A Class I device intended to measure triglyceride (neutral fat) in serum and plasma. Measurements obtained by this device are used in the diagnosis and treatment of patients with diabetes mellitus, nephrosis, liver obstruction, other diseases involving lipid metabolism, or various endocrine disorders.

Triiodothyronine Uptake Test System A Class II device intended to measure the total amount of binding sites available for binding thyroid hormone on the thyroxine-binding proteins, thyroid-binding globulin, thyroxine-binding prealbumin, and albumin of serum and plasma. The device provides an indirect measurement of thyroxine levels in serum and plasma. Measurements of triiodothyronine uptake are used in the diagnosis and treatment of thyroid disorders.

Triose Phosphate Isomerase Test System A Class I device intended to measure the activity of the enzyme triose phosphate isomerase in erythrocytes (red blood cells). Triose phosphate isomerase is an enzyme important in glycolysis (the energy-yielding conversion of glucose to lactic acid in various tissues). Measurements obtained by this device are used in the diagnosis and treatment of congenital triose phosphate isomerase enzyme deficiency, which causes a type of hemolytic anemia.

Trocar A Class I device consisting of a sharp-pointed instrument used in conjunction with a cannula for piercing a vessel or chamber to facilitate insertion of the cannula. In neurology, a trocar is a needle used to puncture an artery prior to catheterization for cerebral angiograms.

Truncal Orthosis A Class II device used to support and/or to immobilize fractures, strains and sprains of the neck and/or trunk of the body. Examples of truncal orthoses are the following: abdominal, cervical, cervicothoracic, lumbar, lumbosacral, rib fracture, sacroiliac, and thoracic orthoses and clavicle splints.

***Trypanosoma* spp. Serological Reagents** Class I devices that consist

200

of antigens and antisera used in serological tests to identify *Trypanosoma* spp. antibodies in a patient's serum. The identification aids in the diagnosis of trypanosomiasis, a disease caused by parasitic protozoans belonging to the genus *Trypanosoma*. Trypanosomiasis in adults is a chronic disease characterized by fever, chills, headache, and vomiting. Central nervous system involvement produces typical sleeping sickness syndrome: physical exhaustion, inability to eat, tissue wasting, and eventual death. Chagas disease, an acute form of trypanosomiasis in children, most seriously affects the central nervous system and heart muscle.

Trypsin Test System A Class I device intended to measure the activity of trypsin (a pancreatic enzyme important in digestion for the breakdown of proteins) in blood and other body fluids and in feces. Measurements obtained by this device are used in the diagnosis and treatment of pancreatic disease.

Tubal Occlusion Device (TOD) A Class III device designed to close the fallopian tube with a mechanical structure such as a band or a clip on the outside of the tube, or a plug or valve on the inside, in order to prevent pregnancy.

Tube (Toynbee diagnostic tube) A Class I listening device intended to determine the degree of openness of the eustachian tube.

Tube (Tympanostomy tube) A Class II device that is intended to be implanted for ventilation or drainage of the middle ear. The device is inserted through the tympanic membrane to permit a free exchange of air between the outer ear and middle ear. A type of tympanostomy tube, known as the malleous clip tube, attaches to the malleous to provide middle ear ventilation. The device is made of materials such as polytetrafluorethylene, polyethylene, silicone elastomer, or porous polyethylene.

Tube (Tympanostomy tube with semipermeable membrane) A Class III device intended to be implanted for ventilation or drainage of the middle ear and for preventing fluids from entering the middle ear cavity. The device is inserted through the tympanic membrane to permit a free exchange of air between the outer ear and middle ear. The tube portion of the device is made of silicone elastomer or porous polyethylene, and the membrane portion is made of polytetrafluoroethylene.

Tube Introduction Forceps A Class II device that is a right-angled forceps used to grasp a tracheal tube and place it in the patient's trachea.

Tweezer-Type Epilator An electrical Class III device intended for hair removal. The device provides a high-frequency electric current at the tip of a tweezer used for removing hair.

U

Ultrasonic Air Embolism Monitor A Class II device used to detect air bubbles in a patient's bloodstream. It may use Doppler or other ultrasonic principle for its operation.

Ultrasonic Diathermy A Class II device for use in applying therapeutic deep heat that applies ultrasonic energy at a frequency beyond 20,000 cycles per second to provide therapeutic deep heat in specific areas of the body. Such tissue heating is used as adjunctive therapy for the relief of pain in selected medical conditions such as muscle spasms and joint contractures.

Ultrasonic Pulsed Doppler Imaging System A Class II device that combines the features of continuous wave, Doppler-effect technology with pulsed-echo effect technology, and is intended to determine stationary body tissue characteristics, such as depth or location of tissue interfaces, or dynamic tissue characteristics, such as velocity of blood or tissue motion. This generic type of device may include signal analysis and display equipment, patient and equipment supports, component parts, and accessories.

Ultrasonic Pulsed-Echo Imaging System A Class II device intended to project a pulsed sound beam into body tissue to determine the depth or location of the tissue interfaces, and to measure the duration of an acoustic pulse from the transmitter to the tissue interface and back to the receiver. This generic type of device may include signal analysis and display equipment, patient and equipment supports, component parts, and accessories.

Ultrasonic Scaler A Class II device used during dental cleaning and periodontal (gum) therapy to remove calculus deposits from teeth by application of an ultrasonically vibrating scaler tip to the teeth.

Ultrasonic Transducer A Class II device applied to the skin to transmit and receive ultrasonic energy. It is used in conjunction with an echocardiograph as an aid in imaging cardiovascular structures. The device includes phased arrays and two-dimensional scanning transducers.

Ultraviolet Activator for Polymerization A Class II device that produces ultraviolet radiation, which is used to polymerize resinous dental pit and fissure sealants or restorative materials by transmission of the light through a rod.

Ultraviolet Detector A Class II device that provides a source of ultraviolet light that is used to identify otherwise invisible material, such as dental plaque, present in or on teeth. Ultraviolet radiation of 320–400 nanometers (nm) is usually innocuous to human skin. However, ultraviolet radiation in the 320–400 nm range can cause erythema and pigmentation in persons naturally susceptible to ultraviolet light and persons ingesting certain drugs or other chemicals that act as photosensitizing agents.

Ultraviolet Lamp for Dermatologic Disorder A Class II device (including a fixture) intended to provide ultraviolet radiation of the body to photoactivate a drug in the treatment of a dermatologic disorder if the labelling of the drug intended for use with the device bears adequate directions for the device's use with that drug.

Ultraviolet Lamp for Tanning A Class I device that is a lamp (including a fixture) intended to provide ultraviolet radiation to tan the skin.

Unipolar Endoscopic Coagulator-Cutter and Accessories A Class II device designed to destroy tissue with high temperatures by directing a high-frequency electrical current through the tissue between an energized probe and a grounding plate. It is used in female sterilization and other operative procedures under endoscopic observation. This generic type of device includes the following accessories: an electrical generator, probes and electrical cables, and a patient grounding plate. This generic type of device does not include devices used to perform female sterilization under hysteroscopic observation.

Untreated Menstrual Pad A Class I device made of an absorbent cotton or synthetic material pad that is used to absorb menstrual or other vaginal discharge and that has not been treated with scent or added drugs or antimicrobial agents.

Untreated Menstrual Tampon A Class II device made of an absorbent cotton or synthetic material plug that is used to absorb menstrual or other vaginal discharge and that has not been treated with scent or added drugs or antimicrobial agents.

Urea Nitrogen Test System A Class II device intended to measure urea nitrogen (an end product of nitrogen metabolism) in whole blood, serum, plasma, and urine. Measurements obtained by this device are used in the diagnosis and treatment of certain renal and metabolic diseases.

Ureteral Stone Dislodger A Class II device that consists of a bougie or a catheter with an expandable wire basket near the tip, a special flexible tip, or other special construction. It is inserted through a cystoscope and used to entrap or remove stones from the lower ureter. This generic type of device includes the metal basket and the flexible ureteral stone dislodger.

Urethral Dilator A Class II device that consists of a specially shaped catheter or bougie and is used to dilate the ureter at the place where a stone has become lodged, or to dilate a ureteral stricture.

Urethrotome A Class II device that is inserted into the urethra and is used to cut urethral strictures and enlarge the urethra. It is a metal instrument equipped with a dorsal-fin cutting blade that can be elevated from its sheath. Some urethrotomes incorporate an optical channel for visual control.

Uretotubal Carbon Dioxide Insufflator and Accessories A Class II device used to test the patency (lack of obstruction) of the fallopian tubes by pressurizing the uterus and fallopian tubes and filling them with carbon dioxide.

Uric Acid Test System A Class I device intended to measure uric acid in serum, plasma, and urine. Measurements obtained by this device are used in the diagnosis and treatment of numerous renal and metabolic disorders, including renal failure, gout, leukemia, psoriasis, starvation or other wasting conditions, and of patients receiving cytotoxic drugs.

Urinary Bilirubin and Its Conjugates (Nonquantitative) Test System A Class I device intended to measure the levels of bilirubin conjugates in urine. Measurements of urinary bilirubin and its conjugates (nonquantitative) are used in the diagnosis and treatment of certain liver diseases.

Urinary Calculi (Stones) Test System A Class I device intended for the analysis of urinary calculi. Analysis of urinary calculi is used in the diagnosis and treatment of calculi of the urinary tract.

Urinary Continence Device (Electrical) A Class III device that consists of a receiver implanted in the abdomen, electrodes for pulsed-stimulation implanted either in the bladder wall or in the pelvic floor, and an extracorporeal, battery-powered transmitter.

Urinary Glucose (Nonquantitative) Test System A Class II device intended to measure glucosuria (glucose in urine). Urinary glucose (nonquantitative) measurements are used in the diagnosis and treatment of carbohydrate metabolism disorders including diabetes mellitus, hypoglycemia, and hyperglycemia.

Urinary Homocystine (Nonquantitative) Test System A Class II device intended to identify homocystine (an analog of the amino acid cystine) in urine. The identification of urinary homocystine is used in the diagnosis and treatment of homocystinuria (homocystine in urine), a heritable metabolic disorder which may cause mental retardation.

Urinary pH (Nonquantitative) Test System A Class I device intended to estimate the pH of urine. Estimations of pH are used to evaluate the acidity or alkalinity of urine as it relates to numerous renal and metabolic disorders and in the monitoring of patients with certain diets.

Urinary Phenylketonuria (Nonquantitative) Test System A Class II device intended to identify phenylketones (such as phenylpyruvic acid) in urine. The identification of urinary phenylketones is used in the diagnosis and treatment of congenital phenylketonuria, which, if untreated, may cause mental retardation.

Urinary Protein or Albumin (Nonquantitative) Test System A Class I device intended to identify proteins or albumin in urine. Identification of urinary protein or albumin (nonquantitative) is used in the diagnosis and treatment of disease conditions such as renal or heart diseases or thyroid disorders, which are characterized by proteinuria or albuminuria.

Urinary Urobilinogen (Nonquantitative) Test System A Class I device intended to detect and estimate urobilinogen (a bile pigment degradation product of red cell hemoglobin) in urine. Estimations obtained by this device are used in the diagnosis and treatment of liver diseases and hemolytic (red cell) disorders.

Urine Collection Bag for Infants A Class I disposable device attached to the infant by an adhesive material and used to collect the infant's urine.

Urine Collector and Accessories A Class II device used to collect urine. The device and accessories consist of tubing, a suitable receptacle, connectors, mechanical supports, and may include a means to prevent the backflow of urine or ascent of infection. This generic type of device includes the corrugated rubber sheath, pediatric urine collector, urinary drainage collection kit, closed urine drainage kit, leg bag, urosheath-type incontinence device, and paste-on device for incontinence.

Urine Culture A laboratory technique used to determine the presence and type of harmful microorganisms in the urinary tract so appropriate treatment may be instituted.

Urine Flow or Volume Measuring System A Class II device that directly or indirectly measures the volume or flow of urine from a patient either during the course of normal urination or while the patient is catheterized. The device may include a drip chamber to reduce the risk of retrograde bacterial contamination of the bladder, a transducer, and electrical signal conditioning and display equipment. This generic type of device includes the electrical urinometer, mechanical urinometer, nonelectric urinometer, disposable nonelectric urine flow rate measuring device, and uroflowmeter.

Urodynamics Measuring System A Class II device used to measure volume and pressure in the urinary bladder when it is filled through a catheter with carbon dioxide or water. The device controls the supply of carbon dioxide or water and may also record the electrical activity of the urinary muscles. The device system may include transducers, electronic signal conditioning and display equipment, a catheter withdrawal device to enable a urethral pressure profile to be obtained, and special catheters for urethral profilometry and electrodes for electromyography. This generic type of device includes the cystometric gas (carbon dioxide), the cystometric hydraulic device, and the electrical recording cystometer, but excludes any device that uses air to fill the bladder.

Urological Catheter A family of Class II devices that include radiopaque urological, ureteral catheter, urethral catheter, coude catheter, balloon retention catheter, upper urinary tract catheter, double-lumen female urethrographic catheter, male urethrographic catheter, and urological catheter accessories.

Urological Catheter (Suprapubic) A Class II device consisting of a flexible tube that is inserted percutaneously through the abdominal wall into the urinary bladder with the aid of a trocar and cannula. It is used to pass fluids to and from the urinary tract. Accessories include catheter and tube, malecot catheter, punch, drainage tube, and suprapubic cannula and trocar.

Urological Clamp for Males A Class II device used to close the urethra of a male to control urinary incontinence, or to hold anesthetic or radiography contrast media in the urethra temporarily. It is an external clamp.

Urological Table and Accessories A Class II device consisting of a table, stirrups, and belts used to support a patient in a suitable position for endoscopic procedures of the lower urinary tract. The table can be adjusted into position mechanically or electrically.

Uroporphyrin Test System A Class I device intended to measure uroporphyrin in urine. Measurements obtained by this device are used in the diagnosis and treatment of porphyrias (primarily inherited diseases associated with disturbed porphyrin metabolism), lead poisoning, and other diseases characterized by alterations in the heme pathway.

V

Vacuum Abortion System (1157) A Class II device designed to transcervically aspirate the products of conception or menstruation from the uterus by using a cannula connected to a suction source. The device is used for pregnancy termination or menstrual regulation. This type of device may include the aspiration cannula, the vacuum source, and the vacuum controller. The Panel includes in this generic type of device those devices identified as "uterine suction cannula," "vacuum abortion unit controller," "vacuum abortion unit source," and "vacuum abortion unit system."

Vacuum-Assisted Blood Collection System A Class I device that uses a vacuum to draw blood for subsequent reinfusion.

Vaginal Douche Kit A Class II device consisting of a bag or a bottle with a nozzle designed to direct a stream of water or solution into the vaginal cavity to cleanse the vagina. The device is not for contraception. A douche kit that includes chemicals or solutions is an over-the-counter vaginal drug product.

Vaginal Insufflator A Class I device used to treat vaginitis by introducing medicated powder from a hand-held bulb into the vagina through an open speculum.

Vaginal Pessary A Class II device consisting of a removable structure placed in the vaginal cavity to support the pelvic organs. It is used to treat such conditions as uterine prolapse (fallen uterus), uterine retroposition (backward displacement of the uterus), and gynecological hernias.

Vaginal Stent (Vaginal dilator) A Class II device designed to completely fill the vaginal cavity in order to enlarge the vagina following reconstructive surgery.

Vancomycin Test System A Class II device intended to measure vancomycin, an antibiotic drug, in serum. Measurements obtained by this device are used in the diagnosis and treatment of vancomycin overdose, and in monitoring the level of vancomycin to ensure appropriate therapy.

Vanilmandelic Acid Test System A Class I device intended to measure vanilmandelic acid in urine. Measurements of vanilmandelic acid obtained by this device are used in the diagnosis and treatment of neuroblastoma, pheochromocytoma, and certain hypertensive conditions.

Varicella-Zoster Serological Reagents Class I devices that consist of antigens and antisera used in serological tests to identify varicella-zoster antibodies in a patient's serum. The identification aids in the diagnosis of diseases caused by varicella-zoster viruses, and provides epidemiological information on these diseases. Varicella (chicken pox) is a mild, highly infectious disease, chiefly of children. Zoster (shingles) is the recurrent form of the disease, occurring in adults who were previously infected with varicella-zoster viruses. Zoster is the response (characterized by a rash) of the partially immune host to a reactivation of varicella viruses present in latent form in the patient's body.

Vascular Clamp A Class II device used to occlude a blood vessel temporarily.

Vascular Clip A Class II implanted device designed to occlude, by compression, blood flow in small blood vessels.

Vascular Grafts (Small bore) A Class III device of less than 6 mm in diameter that is used to replace sections of small arteries. While both woven and knitted dacron and blown PTFE have been used,

Vectorcardiograph

these devices have not performed as adequately as the alternatives for endarterectomy and autogenous vein grafting.

Vectorcardiograph A Class II device used to process and interpret the electrical signal transmitted through ECG electrodes, and to produce a visual display of the magnitude and direction of the cardiac electrical signals.

Vena Cava Clip A Class II implanted device designed to partially occlude the vena cava for the purpose of inhibiting the flow of thromboemboli through that vessel.

Venous Blood Pressure Manometer A Class III device attached to a venous catheter to manometrically indicate the central or peripheral venous pressure.

Ventilator A ventilator is used when artificial respiration must be maintained for a long time. Ventilators operate in different modes: controlled breathing, where ventilators take over all the breathing work; and assisted breathing, where the patient's own spontaneous attempt to breathe causes the ventilator to cycle during inspiration.

Ventilator, Continuous A Class II device used to mechanically control or assist patient breathing. The device may deliver a predetermined percentage of oxygen in the inspired gas. Adult, pediatric, and neonatal ventilators are included in this generic type of device.

Ventilator, Emergency A Class II device that is a demand valve or inhalator used to provide emergency respiratory support through a face mask or catheter inserted into the airway.

Ventilator, External Negative Pressure A Class II device that is a chamber that supports ventilation by using repetitive applications of external negative pressure over the diaphragm and upper trunk.

Ventilator, Manual Emergency A Class II device, usually incorporating a bag and valve, used to provide emergency respiratory support via a face mask or a tube inserted into a patient's airway.

Ventilator, Noncontinuous A Class II device used to deliver intermittently an aerosol to a patient's lungs and/or augment a patient's breathing.

Ventilator, Powered Emergency A Class II device, composed of a demand valve or inhalator, that is used to provide emergency respiratory support via a face mask or a tube inserted into the patient's airway.

Ventilator Tubing A Class II device used as a conduit for gases between the ventilator and the patient during mechanical ventilation of a patient.

Ventricular Assist Devices A Class III device that mechanically

208

helps the right or left ventricle in maintaining proper circulatory blood flow. These devices may be either totally or partially implanted in the body.

Ventricular Bypass (Assist) Devices   A Class III device that mechanically helps the right or left ventricle in maintaining proper circulatory blood flow. These devices may be either totally or partially implanted in the body.

Venturi Mask   A Class II device that contains an air-mixing mechanism used to dilute 100 percent oxygen to a predetermined concentration before delivery to a patient.

Vessel Occlusion Transducer   A Class II device used to supply an electrical signal corresponding to sounds produced in a partially occluded vessel. The device may include motion, sound, and ultrasonic transducers.

Vibratory Cervical Dilator   A Class III device designed to enlarge the cervix by stretching it with a power-driven, vibrating probe head. The device is used to gain access to the uterus or to induce abortion, but is not to be used during labor.

***Vibrio cholerae* Serological Reagents**   Class II devices that are used in the agglutination (an antigen-antibody clumping reaction) test to identify Vibrio cholerae from cultured isolates derived from clinical specimens. The identification aids in the diagnosis of cholera, caused by bacterium Vibrio cholerae, and provides epidemiological information on cholera. Cholera is an acute infectious disease characterized by severe diarrhea with extreme fluid and electrolyte (salts) depletion, and by vomiting, muscle cramps, and prostration. If untreated, the severe dehydration may lead to shock, renal failure, cardiovascular collapse, and death.

Visual Acuity Chart   A Class I device that is a chart, such as a Snellen chart with block letters or other symbols in graduated sizes, intended to test visual acuity.

Visual Field Laser Instrument   An AC-powered Class II device intended to provide visible laser radiation that produces an interference pattern on the retina to evaluate retinal function.

Vitamin A Test System   A Class I device intended to measure vitamin A in serum or plasma. Measurements obtained by this device are used in the diagnosis and treatment of vitamin A deficiency conditions, including night blindness, or skin, eye, and intestinal disorders.

Vitamin B$_{12}$ Test System   A Class II device intended to measure vitamin B$_{12}$ in serum, plasma, and urine. Measurements obtained by this device are used in the diagnosis and treatment of anemias of gastrointestinal malabsorption.

209

Vitamin E Test System   A Class I device intended to measure vitamin E (tocopherol) in serum. Measurements obtained by this device are used in the diagnosis and treatment of infants with vitamin E deficiency syndrome.

Viterous Aspiration and Cutting Instrument   An electrically powered Class II device, which may use ultrasound, intended to remove vitreous matter from the vitreous cavity or remove a crystalline lens.

W

Wall-Mounted Radiographic Cassette Holder   A Class II device that is a support intended to hold and position radiographic cassettes for a radiographic exposure for medical use.

Warmer (Infant radiant)   A Class III device consisting of an infrared heating element placed over an infant to maintain the infant's body temperature by means of radiant heat. The device may contain a temperature monitoring sensor, a heat output control mechanism to regulate the infant's body temperature, and an alarm to alert operators of the device's failure. The device may be placed over a pediatric hospital bed or it may be built into the bed as a complete unit.

Water Circulating Hot or Cold Pack   A Class II device used on body surfaces for heat or cold therapy that operates by pumping heated or chilled water through a plastic bag.

Water Jet Renal Stone Dislodger System   A Class II device used to dislodge stones from renal calyces (recesses of the renal pelvis) by means of a pressurized stream of water through a conduit. The device is used in the surgical removal of kidney stones.

Water Seal Thoracic Drainage System   A Class II device used to restore subatmospheric intrapleural pressure and to drain fluid from the pleural space by means of a chest tube. The device is usually connected to a suction system.

Water Vapor Analyzer   A Class II diagnostic anesthesiology device used to measure the concentration of water vapor in the patient's expired gases by using techniques such as mass spectrometry.

Wax (Intraoral dental)   A Class I device made of wax that is used to construct patterns to customize metal dental prostheses, such as crowns and bridges. In orthodontic dentistry, the device is used to make a pattern of the patient's bite so that crowns and bridges have the proper biting surface contact.

Wheelchair Accessory   A Class I device that is sold separately from the wheelchair and is used for the specific needs of a patient who uses a wheelchair. Examples of wheelchair accessories are the following: armboard, lapboard, pusher cuff, crutch and cane holder, restraint, overhead suspension sling, head and trunk support, blanket, and leg rest strap.

Wheelchair Elevator   A motorized, lifting, Class II device used by a disabled person to move a wheelchair from one level to another.

Wheelchair Platform Scale.   A Class II device with a base designed to accommodate a wheelchair and is used to weigh a person who is confined to a wheelchair.

Whole Blood Hemoglobin Assay   A Class II device consisting of reagents, calibrators, controls, and photometric or spectrophotometric instrumentation used to measure the hemoglobin content of whole blood for the detection of anemia.

Whole Human Plasma or Serum Immunological Test System   A Class I device that consists of the reagents used to measure, by immunochemical techniques, the proteins in human plasma or serum. Measurements of proteins in human plasma or serum aid in the diagnosis of any disease concerned with abnormal level of plasma or serum proteins, e.g., agammaglobulinemia, allergies, multiple myeloma, rheumatoid vasculitis or hereditary angioneurotic edema.

Withdrawal-Infusion Pump   A Class II device designed to accurately inject medications into the bloodstream and to withdraw blood samples for use in determining cardiac output.

Wood's Fluorescent Lamp   A Class I device used to detect fluorescent materials (e.g., fluorescein pigment produced by certain microorganisms) as an aid in the identification of these microorganisms. The device aids in the diagnosis of disease.

Wrist Joint Carpal Lunate Polymer Prosthesis   A one-piece Class II device made of silicone elastomer intended to be implanted to replace the carpal lunate bone of the wrist.

Wrist Joint Carpal Scaphoid Polymer Prosthesis   A one-piece Class II device made of silicone elastomer intended to be implanted to replace the carpal scaphoid bone of the wrist.

Wrist Joint Carpal Trapezium Polymer Prosthesis   A one-piece Class II device made of silicone elastomer or silicone elastomer/polyester material intended to be implanted to replace the carpal trapezium bone of the wrist.

Wrist Joint Metal Constrained Cemented Prosthesis   A Class III device intended to be implanted to replace a wrist joint. The device prevents dislocation in more than one anatomic plane, and consists of either a single, flexible, across-the-joint component or two components linked together. This generic type of device is limited to a device that is made of alloys, such as cobalt-chromium-molybdenum, and is limited to those prostheses intended for use with bone cement.

Wrist Joint Metal/Polymer Semiconstrained Cemented Prosthesis A Class II device intended to be implanted to replace a wrist joint. The device limits translation and rotation in one or more planes via the geometry of its articulating surfaces. It has no linkage across-the-joint. This generic type of device includes prostheses that have either a one-part radial component made of alloys, such as cobalt-chromium-molybdenum, with an ultra-high molecular weight polyethylene bearing surface, or a two-part radial component made of alloys and an ultra-high molecular weight polyethylene ball that is mounted on the radial component with a trunnion bearing. The metallic portion of the two-part radial component is inserted into the radius. These devices have a metacarpal component(s) made of alloys such as cobalt-chromium-molybdenum. This generic type of device is limited to those prostheses intended for use with bone cement.

Wrist Joint Polymer Constrained Prosthesis A Class II device made of polyester-reinforced silicone elastomer intended to be implanted to replace a wrist joint. This generic type of device consists of a single, flexible, across-the-joint component that prevents dislocation in more than one anatomic plane.

Wrist Joint Ulnar (Hemi-wrist) Polymer Prosthesis A mushroom-shaped Class II device made of a medical grade silicone elastomer or ultra-high molecular weight polyethylene intended to be implanted into the intramedullary canal of the bone and held in place by a suture. Its purpose is to cover the resected end of the distal ulna to control bone overgrowth and to provide an articular surface for the radius and carpus.

X

X-ray radiation Therapy System A Class II device intended to produce and control X-rays used for radiation therapy. This generic type of device may include signal analysis and display equipment, patient and equipment supports, treatment planning computer programs, component parts, and accessories.

Xylose Test System A Class I device intended to measure xylose (a sugar) in serum, plasma, and urine. Measurements obtained by this device are used in the diagnosis and treatment of gastrointestinal malabsorption syndrome (a group of disorders in which there is subnormal absorption of dietary constituents and thus excessive loss from the body of the nonabsorbed substances).

Milton Keynes UK
Ingram Content Group UK Ltd.
UKHW040059071024
449327UK00019B/662